I0756848

Other books by Allen R. Remaley

The Hunter Model and its Application in the Teaching of Foreign Languages

A Hint of Jasmine and Lavender: An Erotic Romance

Susquehanna Odyssey

The Teacher's Playbook: A Guide to Success in the Classroom

In the Shadow of Allah

The Awakening of Annie Hill

Letters Late: Things Left Unsaid

Midnight Lullaby: A Tender Tribute to a Woman

Muhammadville

Reflections of a Disgruntled American Gargoyle

The Magician

Ya Should'a Been There

The Tree Climber

Dr. Allen R. Remaley

authorHOUSE

AuthorHouse™
1663 Liberty Drive
Bloomington, IN 47403
www.authorhouse.com
Phone: 1 (800) 839-8640

Published by AuthorHouse 06/19/2020

ISBN: 978-1-7283-6539-8 (sc)
ISBN: 978-1-7283-6538-1 (e)

Library of Congress Control Number: 2020911448

Print information available on the last page.

Any people depicted in stock imagery provided by Getty Images are models, and such images are being used for illustrative purposes only.
Certain stock imagery © Getty Images.

This book is printed on acid-free paper.

DEDICATION

To all those across the world who stood together in unity against a cloaked adversary—COVID-19.

PREFACE

MARCH 18, 2020

This book has to be written. We are at a time in American history when a calamity has struck. A disaster which has the capability of being more threatening than the attack on Pearl Harbor on December 7, 1941, or the collapse of the World Trade Center Towers on September 11, 2001. As of the above date, the United States and, indeed, the world, are faced with a masked death, a virus no one can explain, no one can cure, and no one can know when it might die out.

In this text, no chapter headings will tell the reader when a break has taken place. Like the disease itself, this will be a daily account of what we know at one place in time. Calendar dates will document thoughts and findings about this deadly contagion. My intent is to white-board where we were, what we were doing and what took place before the specter showed itself. It will be a running story of what world leaders, an American President and the people of certain nations did in the face of a world threat.

Others, more schooled, celebrities, elected officials, talking heads from the media, retired Presidents, etc. will sell their accounts of this pandemic. Such writers will have ghost collaborators, editors, proof readers and agents who will help fill the now empty bookstores with stories similar to mine. I don't have time for such things; at my age, my book might remain unfinished, and I do not want my manuscript fingered by some twenty-something year old who just graduated from Yale and who might not remember 9/11. Someone might remember "19", the title of this book.

From where did it come? Did some starving person from some Asiatic country eat a god-awful creature that carried a disease to which only it was immune? Did this thing enter our country from some other nation aboard a container ship and was handled by an unsuspecting stevedore who, because of his physical strength and wellbeing, was not prone to contagion and therefore became an unknown host and carrier of the disease? I don't know. And, by the way, at least by the date of this writing, you don't either.

From the beginning of this pestilence, the media was calling the disease, Coronavirus. Soon, perhaps because of the ease of speaking or the trend of shortening names, we evolved to COVID-19. I like mine, "19". Numbers are easy to remember. They roll off the tongue so readily. People might soon say, "Hey, I've got 19." "Oh, yeah, well, I had it last month. So did my mother. But, she died." Let's drop the humor. The harbinger of death is no joke. Let's talk about what should have been done months ago.

The first detected death from 19 occurred in December 2019, just three months ago in Wuhan, China. The first trial participant in the story of 19 was an American who was repatriated after being quarantined on the Diamond Princess cruise ship docked in Yokohama, Japan in the same month and year. The first presumptive case in the United States was a resident of Oregon in February 2020. Yet, Democrat candidates for the presidency and liberal media never-Trumpers immediately accused the American President of not doing enough to quell the spread of the disease as late as the second week in February, two months after the news of the disease was announced. That trend, in spite of partisan politicking, has quieted down in light of the need for a united front in coping with the virus. Ah, but that, my friends, leads me to ask, "What was Congress and this Nation's Federal Bureau of Investigation doing these last months?" Let's see.

Almost immediately after Donald Trump was elected President, his adversaries began their efforts to discredit his election. From May 2017 through March 2019, the then acting Director of the FBI, Muller, encouraged by Democrats in Congress, began an investigation into whether or not the newly-elected President colluded with Russia in an effort to thwart the Democrat's candidate for the same office. Result? Yep, you guessed it; no collusion, and a complete exoneration. Ah, but, the hatred of the American President was not over.

On December 18, 2019, the Democrat-controlled House of Representatives approved articles of impeachment on charges of abuse of power and obstruction of Congress. A Senate hearing cleared the President of fallacious charges. But, lurking thousands of miles away in China was an insidious infectious disease. And, instead of being aware of such a threat and preparing for the battle to come, Congress, influenced by a liberal media, kept accusing the President of wrong doing.

Before this war record is continued, let me make a declaration concerning my writing. No great effort will be made on my part to ensure that this manuscript is fault free. Should you, the reader, discover a misspelled word, come across a typo, or encounter a questionable grammar point, correct it yourself. Get a dictionary or a thesaurus and add your own comments, but keep it to yourself. A famous movie star once stated in a classic film, "Frankly, my dear, I don't give a damn." My sentiments exactly! Let me add something else.

Friends to whom I have given copies of my other books invariably end up asking me, "Is this book self-published?" They immediately avoid eye contact as if to imply that the book was not authorized by a reputable publishing company. I find that type of criticism amusing knowing full well that their literary output might not fill a sticky note. But, my tongue is held and I even sign the free copy of the text withholding any thoughts about the comment. Let's get on with it.

Today's news coverage, you know, March 19, 2020, shows a renewed and positive effort on the part of local, state and national leaders to encourage such things as social distancing, i.e., refraining from attending gatherings of ten or more people. That is helping; the virus cannot spread if it does not have a welcoming host. The new term, "shelter-in-place" has come up and Governor Cuomo described this as something which might take place during a nuclear attack. Hunkering down might be appropriate. No one has yet suggested getting under a desk. However, the American people are, for the most part cooperating. Oops! "Most" people are together in this war effort. However, our younger generation, our college-age people have been frolicking on American beaches in, yep, large groups. And, it was just reported this morning that the contagion rate of people 20 to 30 has risen over night. While this age group might be able to ward off and recover from the disease, they do become carriers of the rapidly-spreading virus. For our older generation, these young party goers have become walking time bombs. However, my guess is that they, too, will become part of the effort against the invasive malady. But, there are other signs of a growing positivism.

The President is being backed by Congress in authorizing financial aid to families who are not covered by worker's compensation. Talks of helping the travel industry are also taking place. Airlines, cruise ships, trains, buses, hotels and restaurants have taken direct hits. Our efforts in following social distancing, etc. have led to unprecedented unemployment. Mortgage payments, rent payments and credit-card debts have initiated a new worry for many Americans. The government has asked that the American banking system be tolerant in all cases. Let us hope that we are one in this request. My faith in the American way of life tells me that we will see this through as well.

In this morning's briefing by the President, words of

praise were handed out to the American medical profession for its efforts to investigate drugs which might slow, cure or reduce symptoms of the disease. American manufacturing companies are being asked to look into the immediate working up of regulators and respirators so badly needed in hospitals, all of which have too few beds. No one has yet to mention that hundreds of cruise ships are now sitting empty, and that there are thousands of beds available on those ships. I am sure someone smarter than I will bring that up.

Let me say that our American War-Time President is doing a masterful job. He is tirelessly on task and has encouraged the American people to believe in the future. Is he faultless? Of course not. Neither are we. However, President Trump does have the knack of saying things which might be left unsaid. He does not hesitate to remind us that he is doing a great job. And, he does use the term, "China virus". However, in that last slipup, the virus did start in China, not with American soldiers. Get over it, you guys!

Bin to the grocery store lately? Walking through my local supermarket late this morning, meat and fish shelves were empty. On this, my wife's birthday, the market-prepared birthday cakes had disappeared. March 19, must be a popular birthday. Forget toilet paper. Makes me wish Montgomery Wards was still in business (only those who grew up in rural Pennsylvania will understand this). On the drive back to my social-distancing condo, a radio announcement informed me that the State of New York doubled its confirmed cases of 19 overnight. No pickle ball for me today.

Other highlights from today's date are these. The Center for Disease Control has stated that at least 12,000

Americans have died from influenza between October 1, 2019, through February 1, 2020. But that number could rise to 30,000. Remember, this is only the flu, not 19. Fox News just announced that world cases of 19 stand at 236,420. World deaths from the disease are at 9, 800. In the United States, confirmed cases of the virus are at 11,274. Deaths from the virus remain at 157.

Other observations show that fewer deaths from automobile accidents have occurred. However, few people are on the highways. The same could be said about violent crimes; fewer people on the streets, fewer violent crimes. Sequestering and shelter-in-place have made a positive difference. We are being forced to take one day at a time, and we shall see if that helps us win the battle.

Another day, another battle. However, there is both good and bad news. First, the good. Thanks to the electronic media, Americans and others across the world are being updated by the hour on everything from the economy to health. Newspapers, things handled by hundreds of people, seem to be in short supply, and the television and radio coverage have taken up the slack in up-to-date news. Here is just some of the latest.

Both houses of Congress, almost without partisan interference, have joined forces and have proposed stimulus packages designed to keep families in their homes and to put food on their tables. Some squabbling is taking place between Democrat and Republican sponsors of these bills, and I am afraid that it involves whether or not one party or the other receives credit for the proposal. For example, instead of economic stability of household needs, one such proposal had to do with reducing student loans, something which might not be essential at the moment. However, for now, money is being allocated for the immediate relief of basic needs.

Business leaders such as Elon Musk has stated that his automobile company, Tesla, will gear up and consider making respirators badly needed now and in the future. One cruise company has volunteered its ships to be used as floating hospitals where badly needed beds will be available. Jose Andres, a restaurateur, has offered his restaurant chain, World Central Kitchen, as a base of soup kitchens where needy Americans will be fed. In other areas of humanity, there is some good news, too.

President Trump has been seeking the release of Americans held in other countries. One such American hostage has just been given his freedom after being held in Lebanon for several years. Even Iran, Syria and other countries where Americans are being held seem to realize that the threat of 19 might just be the time to become more tolerant. We shall see.

At the present time, Americans are being asked to remain in place. The State of California has just issued a warning that the entire State will be locked down, and that those who do not comply with the shelter-in-place edict will be prosecuted. More and more Americans are heeding the warning, and they are aware of the need to avoid unnecessary contact. That, however, has led to what is being called cabin fever or being cooped up. Some newscasts have reported that playing games and watching movies all day is causing some concern. But, if the case of Anne Frank, a little girl enclosed in an attic for 25 months, we, too, can see this through. The bad news, let's look at it.

Medical professionals have called our attention to smokers and those who vape. Vaping, according to physicians, causes stress to the entire respiratory system, and the majority of those who vape are young people, youth who are more susceptible to contagion and therefore more likely to become carriers of the disease. The next negative case in point is shameful.

Four Senators, three Republicans and one Democrat have been accused of insider trading and selling off their stocks after having had a meeting with the President who stated the prospect of the effects of 19. The meeting took place in January before the threat of the disease became apparent. Those individuals, elected officials in whom we were to give our trust, betrayed the American public. Will they be held accountable? As stated in the novel, **Animal Farm,** "We are all equal, but some are more equal than others."

As of today's date, world figures for those who contracted 19 are at 247, 400. World-wide deaths are at 10, 067. United States figures of those with the disease are 14, 250. U.S. deaths remain at 205. Keep your head down, but remain strong.

MARCH 21, 2020

The latest contamination figures are these: World-wide with the disease is 278, 434. Deaths world-wide are 11, 868. In the United States, 19, 624 carry the virus with 260 American deaths. Americans are still hunkered down. Shutdowns affect movies, shopping malls, libraries, restaurants and non-essential businesses. But, everyday Americans, yes, like me, have been faced with unforeseen hurdles.

A week ago, my physical activity included playing pickle ball six days a week, one hour each morning. In the afternoon, forty minutes on the stationary bike with two-pound weights in each hand pumping as I peddled completed my exercises for the day. What? Did you expect me to use fifteen-pound weights? I'm eighty-one years old, for God's sake. Now, this is where I am now. In pickle ball, at least where I play, thirty or forty people congregate each morning. Common to every one of us is the ball which is handled by each player on each side of the net. Most of us had to adhere to the shelter-in-place advice and avoid contact with so many others. So, back to the gym in the afternoon. Yesterday, on the gym door was a message: "Gym closed due to the COVID-19 threat. Now what?

In the basement of my building, available to all the

residents of this gated community, is a bike storage area. In the past, when I was younger, I would do ten to twenty-mile rides on a men's one-speed old bike. So, dusting off the bike and re-inflating the tires, I dug the old relic out and tried a short ride. Instability from lack of use soon made itself known. It's going to take a readjustment. And, that is the case with all of us. We must adjust to a newness, and most of us are doing just that. But, we have some reluctant dragons among us.

We have seen film clips of the younger college-age generation frolicking on Florida and South Carolina beaches. Our younger generation, used to spring-break traditions, must get in step with the rest of Americans and do their part in avoiding contact and not contaminating others. That is a physical thing. But there is something else which is more odious.

It has already been stated that four Senators, three Republicans and one Democrat, after receiving what amounted to insider trading (advanced briefing on 19), sold off stocks earning them millions of dollars before a drastic drop in the NASDAQ. My immediate thoughts on the matter had to do with an unproven rumor concerning why so many members of Congress suddenly become millionaires. "Oh, come on, Allen, quit complaining!" Oh, that's right, we should not criticize our elected officials…or should we? I think we should, and I think the above four and undisclosed others should be held in contempt and asked to resign. Why not? Other Americans are making a better impression.

The owner of Mission BBQ, an eatery which employs many Americans has a tradition of stopping work at noon every day and playing the National Anthem over a loud speaker and saluting the American flag. A twenty-something girl touched her hand to the window of her grandfather's hospital window to express her delight for having become engaged. Keep it up, Americans. One more observation.

We might have some changing life styles taking shape because of suggested rules. As stated above, my daily exercises have evolved along with that of this 19 thing. This afternoon, after an eight or ten-year hiatus from riding bicycles, I dusted off my old men's single speed, coaster brake heavy metal machine. You know the old adage, "Once you learn how to ride a bike, …". Yeah, that one. Bovine scatology! Tell that to an eighty-one-year-old. Braking, balancing, avoiding other riders and pedestrians, automobiles, etc. took courage. On what turned out to be my shake-down cruise, I took notice of something important. Young adults, some of whom were parents, were doing their own social distancing. Some of the young parents were teaching their children the rules of the road when riding bikes. This more family-like activity might have been brought about by stay-at-home rules governed by this awful virus. When given lemons…

MARCH 22, 2020

Here we go. Another day in which the President and governors from various states will define rules of conduct concerning our battle with 19. The need for ventilators will be outlined, Americans will be reminded that we need to shelter-in-place, continue to use social distance and refrain from overreacting to media reports of empty shelves in supermarkets. The latest figures for those contracting the disease as well as deaths here and abroad will be outlined (today's totals will appear later), and we will receive updates on the medical profession's progress designing a vaccine which might slow or kill the virus. All good stuff. Me? At 3 A.M. I made myself a promise that later, after coffee with Madame, my Christmas lights would be put up on our patio. Huh?

Why not? It will be fun. "Hey, Allen. What are you doing?" "I'm putting up my Christmas lights." "What?" "I'm putting up our Southwest-pepper shaped lights usually displayed in December." "Why?" "Simple. We need to know that a little light will remind people, fellow Americans, that the spirit of working together should be celebrated. What better way than to use a religious reference to encourage everyone to chip in and encourage the feeling of working together. We do not have to refer to the God we worship. That's not the point. However, in the spirit of faith, it will be a visual reminder that some of us are on the front lines… indeed all of us are ready to do anything which might reflect that we have enlisted in the fight."

Who knows what my neighbors might say when they see the red, orange, yellow and green hot-pepper lights on our patio this evening? But my guess is that someone, maybe just one person, will say, "OK, me, too. No, my wife and I do not have millions of dollars to contribute toward the purchase of masks, gloves and ventilators. But we do have spirit. Besides, Christmas lights, Chanukah lights, any lights, might just provide the spark to keep the fires of hope alive. We shall see. But I cannot wait for daylight to help me brighten our patio. Now, back to our front lines.

This morning, New York's Governor Cuomo stated, "We have to come together by staying apart." That statement came after his yesterday visit to New York City parks and playgrounds where he observed crowds of people gathering, playing basketball and socializing. His morning telecast again encouraged people to shelter-in-place. Here in Arizona, people seem to be doing just that. If we are to defeat 19, we must adhere to suggested plans. Some states are in total lockdown.

On the brighter side, one Ohio school district's students recited the Pledge of Allegiance together and then quickly disbanded. Congress is passing bills which would allocate money to those whose mortgages are coming due, help those who have student loans, and aiding small business by providing loans which would help pay employees. One maker of vodka switched gears and began making hand sanitizer and offering 32 oz. free to families who supplied their own containers. One government official stated that before the Coronavirus, Americans were not taking the time to connect with each other. Too busy with their own interests, time was not being taken to reach out to family and friends. Lately, cross-country phone calls are re-establishing family connections. That's a good thing. OK, I will mention this one time, and then I will drop it; could this thing, this all-of-a-sudden scourge, have been an act of God?

Oh, my Christmas lights. Earlier, I finished stringing them up on our patio. Promptly at 4 P.M., shortly before we have our happy hour at our outdoor bar, those lights will come on and remain lighted until midnight. I am sure, our neighbors who walk by…at a distance…will ask, "Getting ready for Easter?" My response will be, "No, but the thought is good. Just our way of saying, 'Hi, neighbor. We're with you.' Tomorrow, I hope to report on my neighbors' comments.

Earlier today, Governor Cuomo of New York reported that price gauging was going on, something Americans encounter during catastrophic events. Sanitary masks which had been selling for $.80 are now selling for $7.00 since every state in the union is competing for medical supplies. Cuomo also predicted that 40 to 80 percent of New York State residents will come down with the dreaded 19.

Today's figures for world-wide infections from the disease are at 329, 080. Deaths across the globe are at 14, 376. Americans contaminated from the disease are at 32,080. Deaths are at 400.

MARCH 23, 2020

There is a steady increase in contagion of the 19 virus. Today's figures world-wide are at 350, 536, compared to yesterday's 329, 140. World-wide deaths today are at 15,328 compared to yesterday's 14,376. In the United States, those who contracted the disease are at 35,225 compared to yesterday's 32.080. Deaths in the U.S. today are at 471, compared to yesterday's 400. Reasons for such increases include young people not heeding the shelter-in-place advice from state and federal authorities as well as the inability to totally understand the disease itself. However, here in Arizona, there seems to be adherence to suggested ways of dealing with the sickness.

Yesterday, I related the story of installing Christmas lights on our patio. Promptly at 4 P.M., those lights came on, and Madame et moi took up our stations at our outdoor-patio bar. Passersby, some outfitted in masks, looked on, but could not utter any words of encouragement or disbelief; cloth-covered mouths do prevent communication. However, on patios next to ours, neighbors came out and expressed their positive opinions of what they recognized as an attempt to inspire togetherness and hope. From distances of twenty to forty feet, we exchanged sincere greetings and expressions of unity. Everyone offered assistance if and when needed, we shared some levity about toilet-paper hoarding, and we all agreed that there was solidarity in isolation. We will probably do the same later on today.

In what seemed to be negative news, news accounts reported that Congress, both houses, could not agree on passing a bill concerning economic relief for individuals, small and large business. The ugly head of politics rises out of its shelter and calls for such things as reducing college loans to every student to the tune of $10,000. The Senate had proposed that no college loan payments would be required for three months. For politicians wishing to attract the praise of those in debt for such loans, grandstanding took the podium. I wonder how many students who were at Florida and South Carolina beaches last week used some to their college loan money to pay for play. Enough of that. We are at war. Let's get back to the battlefield.

There are still some stories battlefront heroes. One wood-working shop is making tables for use by home-schooled students and small children. The tables which can be turned into work desks are offered at no cost, and they come in pieces which are put together in the home. Automobile companies have offered to retool their plants in order to build ventilators badly needed by those who contract 19. So, while there are reluctant dragons among us, most Americans are united, and because of that, our country will remain strong. But there is always that ten percent who never get the word.

This morning, in the halls of Congress, a bill was brought before the Senate which, if passed, would have provided badly-needed funds for unemployment benefits, hospital supplies, income for those who do not qualify for certain benefits, money for mortgage and rent payments, etc. That money is needed immediately. However, the virus and partisan politics have deprived fellow Americans of the ammunition needed to continue the battle. Five Republicans have contracted the virus and have removed them because of social distancing from the voting. Democrats, realizing that they now had the majority in the Senate, held up the bill's passing because they wanted to add a provision which would have protected and encouraged union membership among American workers—something not crucial to what is immediately needed. Chuck Schumer, minority leader in the Senate encouraged his party to vote against the bill before the Senate. Mitch McConnell, the majority leader had a verbal dispute with his opponents, and the bill has not yet passed. Such grandstanding and political tongue wagging is not needed, and it smacks of a shameful display disdain for the American public. Enough said.

In more positive news, a priest in Connecticut gave last rites to a dying Coronavirus patient via a telephone hookup with family and friends. Unable to gather at the hospital bed, a phone was held to the ear of the dying man, and family and friends were able to say their goodbyes. Humanity still reigns in some places.

Update: As of 1:54 M.T., Congress still has not passed the bill intended to bolster the economy. Can't wait until November 2.

Yesterday, a few minutes before my daily bike ride, one of my neighbors was coming in the door of our building. He had just completed his morning walk, said hello and sat down in one of the chairs in the foyer. We exchanged verbal greetings (no handshakes here), asked about family health and almost immediately, our conversation evolved into the virus and its complications.

Now, my neighbor is a resident of a mid-western state. He is a college-educated, hard-working contractor running a company whose workers could either build, repair, renovate, relocate or tear down your existing home. He is a solid red, white and blue American who strongly believes in his country and its President. I value his opinion, so I asked him what he thought of the present lock down, the pandemic and our life as it has changed. I was not ready for his answer; too caught up in the efforts by local, state and national efforts to quell this pestilence, I expected him to reply saying that we, the American people, were coping as best we could. But, when he said, "In my opinion, I think all this is some kind of conspiracy.", I wanted to hear more.

Oh, OK, don't tell me that you or someone close to you has not brought up the idea that someone, some country, some evil scientist or some power-hungry overly-rich person has collaborated with or, yes, colluded with another party to cause havoc in the world. Sure you have! You might not voice that opinion yourself, but I'll bet you questioned the F.B.I. investigation and the impeachment process thinking…*Man, there are some haters of the American President and how well things seem to be going.* Sure you did! Is the idea of plotting or scheming so out of place? Intrigued by my neighbor's quick answer to my question, I wanted to hear more.

From my neighbor's comments, I was able to gather that he believed that there were still a lot of "never-Trumpers" in the mix. He further added that while the source of the contagion might not be the Democrats, billionaires such as George Soros, Mike Bloomberg and others might have gotten together and encouraged the development of a plague-like virus which could take down the economy and destroy the American President. Russia's president was mentioned, the nation of China was suspect since it was the geographical origin of the virus…in spite of the American media's accusation of racism regarding the President's calling the bug the "China virus". He, this American caught up in the social distancing and the other cautionary "in-place" suggestions, also suggested that science had played a role in this war on people and nations. Could some germ have been invented which would reduce world population and change life as we knew it? As if China was again behind the virus, it was mentioned that China could afford to lose half its population and still survive as a world leader. As if anything else would cause concern, one might ask what has happened with the student protests in Hong Kong. No one seems to mention that. Hum? Speculation? How do I know?

As of today, Congress is still acting like school-yard bullies by holding up the vote on a bill which would provide some stability to working Americans and help increase badly-needed medical supplies. The inability to work in a bipartisan way and promote the general welfare of the nation is like waving the white flag of surrender to a military adversary. In this day and time, that hesitancy to provide immediate help borders on treason. But, let's throw a little light on all this.

In New York City yesterday, a young couple got married on the sidewalk of a city street while bystanders remained the customary six feet apart. The marriage was officiated by a friend from a fourth-floor window just above the newly-married couple. Ford Motor Company, 3M, GE and other industries have changed operations and have begun making sanitary masks, gowns, ventilators and respirators. A pizza maker took out a $50, 000 loan to make sure his employees were paid during the closing down period. In this comedic two-mask scenario, these positive examples of the American spirt are in contrast to the sad face of Congress.

World-wide figures of contagion are at 392,380. Deaths are at 17,159. U.S. contagion is at 46,480. Deaths are at 593.

Activity around our patio last evening was brisk, full of hope, and even toilet paper was discussed. Don't ask me why. On that subject, what is the fascination with this round tube of tissue? Lately, and since the beginning of the Coronavirus scare, all sorts of paper products have become scarce. The butt of jokes and barroom humor, toilet tissue and other paper products might now be part of the changes taking place across America. We might be headed for our own 'Back-to-the-Future' mentality.

Unless you are a farmer or grew up in rural America like me, toilet paper was not an item which held much value, and we did not see shelves of this precious commodity on grocery shelves. Living with my grandmother in a backwoods community of Pennsylvania, I got used to a two-holer, a sturdily-built outhouse inside of which, on a seated platform, ran a wide, wooden board with two appropriately-sized holes. Smelly and fly-infested in the summer, freezing cold in the winter, the occupant wasted little time taking care of business. Toilet paper? No way! Montgomery Ward and Sears-Roebuck catalogues served two purposes—reading material and, well, you know the other. Each catalogue lasted for nearly a year, and the following year's replacement was eagerly awaited by both readers and needers. And, the hole itself? Every two or three years, we would dig a six-foot deep and four-foot wide pit, and relocate the outhouse over top of this new space. Lots of lime would be used before backfill was added to the old, do I dare say, "dump"?

Paper towels have also gone missing lately from grocery shelves. Something tells me that Americans will soon be using old towels to sop up spills and then deposit them along with the laundry. Saves time and money. Paper plates might soon become a thing of the past. Using ceramics, dishes reserved for holidays and special occasions might reappear on the nation's tables. Change is sometimes a good thing, and there is no doubt that 19, that invisible scourge, is changing America.

MARCH 25, 2020

Before any observations of daily life take place, these are the latest reports concerning contagion and deaths: Worldwide confirmed of those who have contracted 19 are at 436,139. Deaths are at 19,648. In the United States, 55,238 are infected. Deaths are at 802. Yes, there is an increase and one which should be watched closely.

This morning's news, concerning American business, is not good. Clothing stores and big-box shoe sales are suffering since most those establishments are closed. The prognosis seems to point to the fact that buying clothing will, should this malady end, will not see the levels of purchases of the past. Will women wear dresses? Will men wear suits? We shall see. But there is more evidence that things have changed.

Yesterday, after an automobile trip to a library in an effort to return reading and listening material, as you might expect, that library was closed. No problem. The outdoor book return slots were available. Mission accomplished, and no contact with library personnel was necessary. Returning to my underground garage, I was waved down by a neighbor leaving the complex. She called my attention to the fact that one of my headlights was out (I have one of those cars on which the lights are constantly working while in drive).

From a distance, I thanked my helpful neighbor, and immediately called my VW service department. This took place at 7:45 A.M.

My call was immediately answered, and I was told that a replacement bulb could be done. I was pleased; my VW center is one of the busiest in Scottsdale, and a lot of upscale autos are serviced there. No, not mine. I have a 2002 VW Cabrio…44,000 actual miles, and it does not qualify as an upscale-automobile. When I asked when my repair might take place, the service manager said, "How soon can you get here?" Fifteen minutes later, I was pulling in to the service department, an area which was completely devoid of other cars and customers. No one was waiting in line for either service or sales.

A service employee met me at the door, inquired about my needs, and minutes later, my automobile was pulled into the empty service bays. As a precaution, I requested that both bulbs for my headlights be replaced, a job which I was informed would take about thirty minutes. So, I took a seat in the customer waiting area…alone. No other customers, either for repair or those interested in sales, appeared. Around 9 A.M., sales personnel started to arrive and made themselves busy waiting for potential customers. None arrived. Why this short observation? Easily answered; our lives will change abruptly in the coming months. The penchant for new shoes, new clothing, automobiles, ocean cruises, and trips abroad will diminish. And, yes, so will our economy.

As this allegory is put on record, the federal government

is contemplating passing a Coronavirus Relief Bill. The Senate and House of Representatives now have such a bill before them, a bill which would infuse the economy with badly-needed funds to the tune of $2 trillion dollars. I don't know how many zeroes that entails; I deal in hundreds, not trillions. But there is a catch. In spite of the fact that Americans now unemployed need money for mortgage payments, rent payments, food purchases and the payment of credit-card bills, the stimulus bill has not been passed and forwarded to the President for signature. Why? There are those in the House of Representatives who want to use the crisis to include in the bill's offerings such things as the encouragement of union support, the paying off of student loans, and the inclusion of incentives for green environmental legislation, and none of these things are crucial to our survival. Partisan politics has raised its ugly head once again. One of the Senators said yesterday that "Those who have been holding up the bill's signing should have their head in a bag." Maybe so. At this very moment, 9:15 A.M., Mountain Time, the Leader of the Senate just announced that the bill will be passed...after three days being held up.

On the medical scene, many physicians are advocating that the same drug used for malaria eradication, Hydroxychloroguine, or Chloroquine, be used in experimenting with slowing the virus and its infection of others. Oops! Factions of the medical profession want a more scientific approach where trials will be evaluated before the drug can be said safe. It is ironic that the above drug can be prescribed by any doctor to those who ask for it. If I contract 19, I would...Ah, Hell, you decide.

In other news, the Tokyo Olympics have been postponed until 2021 or longer. Four thousand ventilators have been sent to New York City, and New York's Governor is calling for more suggesting that President Trump put into effect the Federal Defense Production Act. Politics again? Don't accuse me of such a suggestion. I'm just a bystander, but I still see, hear and sometimes think. Who was that Frenchman who said, *"Je pense, donc je suis."*? I wonder what that means.

MARCH 26, 2020

Before this chronicle of American life and the war on Coronavirus continues, let me bring you up to date on current figures for contamination and death world-wide and in the United States. One week ago, on March 19, world-wide numbers infected with the disease were at 236,420. Deaths across the globe numbered 9,800. On that same date in the United States, 11,274 were infected. U.S. deaths were at 157. In stark contrast are today's figures. World-wide infections are at 487, 648. Deaths are now at 22,030. On March 26, in the United States, infections are at 69,197, and deaths are at 1,046. In the United States, in a one-week period, total infections and deaths have increased 16%, a catastrophic figure which is stressing government, industry and citizenry. World-wide figures are worse. And, what is Congress doing about it? Here we go.

Over a week ago, the Coronavirus Stimulus Bill was in discussion and was to be brought before the Senate for passage under a Republican majority. In steps the virus, and five Republican Senators contracted the virus thus giving the Democrats the majority in the Senate. At the same time, the Speaker of the House, Nancy Pelosi, had drafted and inserted new proposals to be included in the bill. What proposals, you ask? Millions of dollars were to be included for the Endowment for the Arts, Howard University was to receive millions for education benefits, etc. Most of these last-minute insertions had nothing to do with the plight of the American worker. As of today, Thursday, a bill which would provide relief for the American people is still not passed. OK, tell me that partisan politics does not harm our citizens. Wait! That will depend on your political affiliation…won't it.

Two trillion dollars have been designated to go to needy American families. I can't even imagine the number of zeroes in that figure. As stated previously, I deal in ten's and hundreds, not trillions. But we are already seeing the effect on American business. On a bike ride yesterday, I encountered a friend and his wife along the bike path. They were sitting on a park bench taking a rest. I placed myself on the other side of the path (social distancing) and said, "Look up at the sky. Tell me what you see." Now, the shy in AZ is usually clear blue…unless you have a haboob, the Arizona dust storm. My friends responded, "We nothing." I said, you're right. No vapor trails. No planes are flying. Outside our building, no private jets are flying into the airport at Scottsdale. The drone of private jets carrying corporate officers is but a memory. All quiet on the Southwestern front.

Let's jump back to the increasing numbers of affected humans and the reasons for such an increase in contagions. We have been told repeatedly to shelter-in-place and to abide by social distancing. However, there is always that ten percent who never get the word as well as those who say, "I cannot stay away from my grandchildren." Maybe so, but some recent events can explain what happened in

Italy, Spain, New Orleans and London. In Italy, a country dedicated to the clothing industry, it is rumored that much of the high-end clothing is done in China and that many Chinese are employed in clothing factories in Italy. Those employees travel home for holidays. In Spain, a recent soccer match had thousands jammed together in stadiums across that country. In New Orleans, huge crowds at Mardi Gras helped spread the virus. London, like New York City, attracts tourists. Yesterday, in the U.K., Parliament shut down completely. About time. Such large gatherings have come to an end. But there is good news, too.

On March 29, Elton John is hosting a T.V. special called the Living Room Concert, a commercial-free event with no audience other than those in their living rooms. Many Americans are showing their patriotism by flying flags, putting up holiday lights and adhering to recommended warnings about congregating in big groups. Now, if we could get our elected representatives to join in the war effort, all might be well. There will always be detractors.

Yesterday, New York State's Governor Cuomo complained, rightfully so, about the lack of respirators and other hospital needs. One of the things which seemed to be lacking were hospital gowns. Huh? The hospital gown, at least most of them, is made up of cotton fabric that can withstand repeated laundering in hot water. What? No washing machines in hospitals? Get some!

One last admonition. In this run-on chronicle, mistakes are going to be made. You have already been warned about that. If repetitions are made, think of them as tracer rounds; they will let you know where the fire is coming from. As far as the mistakes go, correct them. Gives you something to do.

Another day, another increase in confirmed infections and deaths. World-wide for those having the virus is 551,337. Deaths are at 24,863. The United States now has the largest number of those infected at 86,012, a figure higher than any other country in the world. U.S. deaths are at 1,301. New York State has the most infected people. However, Louisiana is increasing in confirmed cases, and Mardi Gras is being blamed for the increasing outbreaks. The fallout from the disease is taking its toll across America.

Opening day for the American baseball season has been postponed. The U.S. Open golf tournament will not take place, and Southwest Airlines is cancelling 1,500 flights per day. The U.S. Stock Market is languishing at dangerously-low levels. And, to the dismay of the American public and to its frustration with Congress, the Coronavirus Relief Package has not yet been passed. Several members of both houses of Congress are holding out because of what seems to be pet projects. In the meantime, Americans who would benefit from the bill's passage are waiting for funds needed for everything from food purchases to rent and mortgage payments. In my opinion, the time has come for term limits for members of Congress, men and women whose income is not in jeopardy. Shameful exhibition of political partisan politics. Unforeseen occurrences have taken place.

On two of America's aircraft carriers, the USS Theodor Roosevelt and the USS Ronald Reagan, at least thirty crew members have taken ill with the virus. Those ships will soon pull into ports, and those weapons, vital to American security, will be temporarily taken out of service. Conspiracy theory? It is interesting to note that a virus, conceived by means unknown, has shut down not only the American economy, but it has also altered our ability to defend ourselves. Coincidence? Your guess.

In what has recently become a social trend, the habit of vaping, the use of electronic cigarettes, has had repercussions. Vaping does have a harmful effect on the human lung. The virus, this 19, is a respiratory disease and therefore requires ventilators and respirators, both of which remain in short supply. Smoking, especially by the younger generation, is not an attractive thing. But Americans are still doing some good things.

Social distancing, sheltering-in-place and avoiding even close family contact is practiced. Those walking by our patio, wave and say hello at a distance. Will such practices slow the progress of this disastrous evil affliction? Time will tell. However, there is a call and a need for Americans to get back to work. Part of this desire comes from the fact that people need to feel productive. Much of the desire is the simple fact that our economy is in need of a jump start. After all, how will we pay for representation in Congress?

MARCH 28, 2020

Ah, the weekend. Good news and bad. So, let's go. World-wide figures of those testing positive for 19 are over 600,000. Deaths are at 28,000. U.S. counts for those testing positive are at 100,000; deaths are at 1,600. Both areas show high rates of increase, and there seems to be no slowdown of climbing totals. Will spring weather help reduce contagion? Let us hope.

Efforts to ease the pressure for more hospital beds and supplies show promise. The American military hospital ships, the USNS Comfort will soon pull into New York City today, and the USNS Mercy will arrive in Los Angeles shortly. Both ships will supply hundreds of beds and support personnel. The United States Corps of Engineers will build temporary hospitals in areas across the country where needed. Supplying those structures with trained care givers will be a problem. Some medical schools are graduating students early to help ease the short supply of medically-trained personnel. The problem of equipping those health-care people remains a problem.

The 3M manufacturing company has agreed to make surgical masks badly needed in epicenter areas such as New York City and Louisiana. Ah, but there is a catch. Suppliers of these masks, once they receive shipments from 3M, have been price gauging for these products. Mark Cuban, the owner of the Dallas professional basketball team recently suggested that 3M should warn their suppliers that they could lose the franchise of selling company products. I would suggest something a little stronger. It might indeed be time for President Trump to invoke the War-Time Powers Act. Why not? However, no matter what moves are made to ease the situation, there will always be criticism from all sides of the aisle…depends on whom you voted for…don't it.

Other good news? The Coronavirus Relief Bill passed by Congress was signed yesterday, and badly-needed funds will be distributed across the country in the next few weeks. Some political grandstanding took place during the above process, but the bill will help both individuals and industry to weather the storm for a short time. American workers now in shutdown will still receive some money to ease the cost of living. As the American President continues to say, "It wasn't their fault." He's right. This virus in an equal-opportunity killer. Will he, the responsible person in office be criticized for his input? Of course; our political parties will make sure of that.

The relief bill did have some questionable riders. Providing money for the Endowment for the Arts, increasing the amount of funds to Planned Parenthood, and encouraging the membership in workers' unions might need scrutiny. Oh, well, politicians will be politicians. There is no doubt that Americans are volunteering to fight on the front lines against this plague. Mike Lindell, the inventor of MyPillow, has retrofitted one of his buildings and is now making hospital supplies and offering them at reduced prices to healthcare centers. And, there is cause for hope among those seeking vaccines and virus-control drugs.

The drug, hydroxychloroquine, used in quelling malaria has been suggested as something which can ease the symptoms of the 19 infection. Used in conjunction with Z-pack, the evidence of lessening the effects of the virus is promising. If governmental requirements for testing new drugs is reduced, such a procedure might be successful. The above drugs are already approved for related illnesses. Getting approval for their immediate use should be no problem

The American people are resilient, and they want to get back to work. Work ethic in this country is one of the things which has made Americans strong. Belief in family and friends is another, and that leads me to cite another phenomenon. Americans have been asked to shelter-in-place and to use social distancing. Knowing that such suggestions were given near the end of February, my guess is this: get ready for a lot of December babies.

MARCH 29, 2020

And, the forward progress of 19 marches on. Overnight, world-wide figures of positive cases of the virus are at 661,000, 60,000 more than yesterday. World-wide deaths from the disease are now at 31,700, and increase of almost 4,000. In the United States, 24,000 more infected people brought the total to 124,000. Deaths rose 500 to a total of 2,100. Without practicing sheltering-in-place and social distancing, the above figures would most likely be off the charts. There is new information that might cut increases.

Yesterday, a New York City physician gave a Fox News update on how the virus is transmitted to other people. The use of face masks by those other than healthcare workers was downplayed. The doctor emphatically pointed out that we get infected from our hands. No physical contact with others was emphasized. Anytime we touch anything or anyone, we are in danger of becoming infected. Should contact take place, we are asked to wash our hands thoroughly and, in no circumstances should we touch our face. The disease is transmitted by hand to our eyes, nose and mouth. We have been asked to shrink our social circle, and that includes family members. Wash your hands often, don't touch people or things, and if you do, cleanse self and things touched.

Social distancing includes making only essential trips (grocery stores, pharmacies, refueling automobiles). Another warning was issued concerning what might be termed a panic move.

Federal and state safety personnel have noticed that there is a run on gun stores in an effort to purchase weapons. The primary danger is that most of those seeking weaponry are those without any official training in gun safety. Individuals without any knowledge of the proper handling of weapons often leave them in plain view. When confined in close quarters, accidents will occur, emotions will be high, and unfortunate deaths could occur. Should we quell the virus, something else will occur. People will want to get rid of their guns, and in the haste to return to normal, guns at a reduced price will fall into the wrong hands.

In an effort to throw more light on the present crisis, I decided to search out more information on the common flu, something people encounter every season (November through May). Last evening, during a social-distancing discussion with friends (less than six), I asked those around me (six feet away), what they thought the number of deaths from the common flu was in 2019. Most people responded by suggesting between 6 and 10 thousand. I was surprised to learn that 80,000 Americans died last year from that disease. The Coronavirus is supposedly more lethal. The CDC in Atlanta stated that last year's influenza outbreak was the highest total for the disease in the last four decades. Not good news. I hate research.

Every so often, I wonder if we are living an episode of 'The Twilight Zone', and I expect Rod Serling to step up and predict some terrible scenario involving the Earth's efforts to rid itself of nasty things. We have fewer planes in the air, fewer automobiles on our highways, and fewer people doing those things which put contaminants in the air. Are these viruses the Earth's way of reducing the threat of its destruction? Impossible, Serling has been dead for many years. Let's jump to the positive.

At 9 P.M. Eastern, Elton John will host a concert with no audience but those at home watching television. This music fest, an effort to bring something bright in all this darkness, will perhaps steel us to remain strong in the face of this war-like threat. I hope they include a few banjo pieces in the mix. Maybe "Camptown Races".

Overnight, Coronavirus figures jumped again. World-wide, contagion spiked to 737,929, almost 100,000 over yesterday. Deaths soared to 35,019, 4,000 increase since March 29. In the United States, confirmed cases rose to 143,055, 20,000 over the day before. U.S. deaths were almost 400 more at 2,513. Frightening figures for all Americans. A leading WH doctor predicted that more than 100,000 Americans could die from 19, the unforgiving pandemic.

In an effort to bring some light and music to the American public without bringing people to large-venue areas, Elton John hosted the Iheart Family Concert for Americans. Last night at 9 P.M. Eastern, various artists performed from their living rooms in a live broadcast over Fox News and other networks. Now, look, I am not in any way qualified to evaluate the above effort to bring smiles to American faces. However, instead of well-known artists, a group of lesser-seen musicians sang a medley of their hit. One young man strummed his guitar and sang while chewing his gum, a feat that few might be able to achieve. The others? Let's just say that most Americans went to bed without much enthusiasm for modern-day music. Did I contribute to the many requests for funds via the Internet?

Yes, but my meager contribution will probably not bring much help to food kitchens and health-care workers. Total contributions during the event are not yet available.

Two U.S. Navy hospital ships pulled into ports, one in New York City and another in Los Angeles. Both ships are equipped with twelve operating rooms and medical personnel. In Central Park in New York, the Army Corps of Engineers constructed at least ten makeshift hospital tents providing at least a thousand beds for those who will need them. Did certain Americans express their appreciation for the effort to reduce the suffering? Some did. Some did not. The American Speaker of the House, Nancy Pelosi, quipped, "His (the President') delaying of getting equipment to where it is needed is deadly. As the President fiddles, people are dying." American media, a four-year foe of the elected official in the White House, echoed the Speaker's criticism. Such a negative stance cannot go unanswered.

While the majority of those in Congress, both Democrat and Republican, approve of the Administration's efforts to fight the virus and its complications, the meanness and political bias dampen the American spirit of cooperation in this fight. It appalls me how grown men and women in the media and in the Halls of Congress have allowed their partisan bickering to hinder a common-front effort in our fight to eradicate a military, medical and economic threat to our Nation. Such behavior borders on what small children might do when they do not get their way. Screaming, accusing elected officials of putting American lives in jeopardy smacks of something puerile, and it puts a stain on our ability to remain united. Shame on the retractors and their silliness at such times in history.

On the other side of the coin, we have some supporters of the American effort and the American President. This morning on Fox News, journalists asked pertinent questions of the President. They did not question Administration efforts to ease suffering. They did not question the President's recommendation of extending the closedown of business and stay-at-home procedures. One young female journalist expressed her sentiments by saying that she and others would offer prayers for the President and his success in bringing the virus to its end. Weeks ago, Nancy Pelosi said that she, too, would pray for the President indicating the perhaps his mental health was in question. Nice, Nancy! Very cute and childlike.

Let's end this day on the positive. The Coronavirus Relief Package has been signed and within two weeks, checks will be forwarded to needy Americans designed to keep them safe for up to ten weeks. The anti-malaria drug, Hydroxychloroquine, is now being used in 1100 cases in New York City on those who tested positive for 19. This is being done without long, drawn-out examination of results. The final chapter on the drug's use might prove positive. Let's pray (oh, there's a word) that it is.

How do I begin today's commentary? Should I be despondent, depressed, down in the mouth? Hell, I don't have time for that; there is too much good in our world, too many Americans willing to join the fight in this war against what we are calling COVID-19. I call it "19". Whatever its name, it is insidiously lethal, and it must be killed. Let's look at current levels of contagion and death.

World-wide infections rest at 800,048. Deaths are at 38,714. Both numbers are up from yesterday. In the United States, positive cases for the virus are at 164,610 and deaths at 3,170. Numbers here are up as well. However, efforts across the Nation are being made to quell and slow the spread of the contagion.

At yesterday's White House briefing, it was reported that American industry is stepping up efforts to help where needed. Ford Motor Company and GE Health Care manufacturing are entering into a joint effort to design and construct ventilators, and a Ford representative reported that 5,000 ventilators would be produced in the next 100 days. Proctor and Gamble has worked with United Technologies to provide sanitizing agents. Mike Lindell from MyPillow has changed one of his production buildings into a mask-making facility. The list goes on, and this united effort is a source of inspiration to the American people. Johnson & Johnson predicted that its company would produce a vaccine against the virus by September of this year. But, there is more.

Yesterday, neighbors from our New York residence called to inquire about the health of our health. My wife and I thanked them. Our fellow residents of our gated community here in AZ dropped by and offered to pick up groceries and, of course, the American specialty, pizza. That, too, is an on-going indication of at-home help. However, my wife and I are just a little over 80 years old, and we will decline further offers of help. After all, we do not need either walkers or oxygen tanks. And, Hell, I ride my one-speed bike at least one hour a day before I collapse at happy hour.

On the home front and in many communities, drive-through testing areas are now available to those wishing to confirm positive or negative results of the test. President Trump announced yesterday that a new testing machine has been developed which gives results in less than fifteen minutes. In the weeks to come, Americans will begin to receive monetary assistance in the form of checks which will help them in the coming months. Are there still problems? Huh? Let's see.

A Holland America cruise ship is now resting of the coast of Florida requesting a docking at Fort Lauderdale. On board, dozens have flu-like systems and four people aboard that ship have died. The Governor of Florida, Ron DeSantis, is reluctant to allow the cruise ship to dock. He is worried about his fellow Floridians. Why wouldn't he be? His decision might be influenced by what Dr. Birx,

White House Coronavirus Response Coordinator, reported yesterday. She predicted that the United States could see as many as 200,000 deaths in the months to come. Her colleague, Dr. Anthony Fauci, projected that U.S. deaths could range from 1.6 to 2.2 million in a worst-case scenario. That, my fellow Americans, is almost too terrible a cost. One death, as uttered the President, is too many. Is there more negative news. Depends on your political persuasion. If you are the Speaker of the House of Representatives driven by progressive colleagues, you will constantly criticize the American President. If you are the Governor of the State of New York, you will constantly criticize the federal government of not reacting quickly enough. *Plus ca change, plus c'est la meme chose.* I wish I knew what that meant. Let's see what takes place during the rest of this day.

OK, there is one last thing. On my bike ride today, it was hard to overlook the fact that, nature, in the midst of all this, continues on as usual. While there are few people out on the trails, animals, humming birds, quail, woodpeckers and other birds of the Southwest, are building nests and caring for their young. Ground squirrels and other rodents are scurrying about gathering food. Rattlesnakes, although I have not come across them yet, are leaving their dens in search of the same scurrying ground squirrels. Oblivious of the plague now invading the human realm, nature's innocence is abounded. A sign of life to come?

COVID-19 has been eradicated! April fool's! Today in French-speaking countries, people of all ages are sneaking up on family and friends and secretly attaching paper fish to their backs. This April 1 tradition has lent humor to the first day of April since Henri IV in the sixteenth century. Today, across the world, pranks are no longer considered in vogue, and today's virus counts tell us why. Across the world, 878,767 people have become infected and 43,260 have died. These figures represent an increase of 78,000 positive and 5,000 dead in one day. Figures in the United States are similar. Positive contractions are at 189,753 with over 4,000 dead. Compared to yesterday's figures, over 20,000 more people have tested positive and almost 1,000 more people have died within a span of twenty-four hours. The news does not get any better.

Dr. Birx, the WH Coordinator of our fight against this insidious disease tells us that unless we hold fast to our shelter-in-place directives, Americans could see as many as 200,000 deaths in a best-case scenario. Dr. Anthony Fauci, Birx's colleague, projects that U.S. deaths could range from 1.6 million to 2.2 million in a worst-case comparison. President Trump just called for a continuation of our stay-at-home procedures through April 30. Reference to efforts to contain the virus has been called, "mitigation". This effort, following directions, social distancing, staying at home, will perhaps take the edge off, i.e. mitigate the situation. Let us hope.

In the meantime, America's military might has also been affected. The USS Theodore Roosevelt, one of our Nation's aircraft carriers, has pulled into Guam with over 300 of its personnel testing positive for the virus. A skeleton crew remains on board to make sure the nuclear reactors are working. It is interesting to note that it was not a missile which put our floating weapon out of commission, it was a microscopic bug. This same infestation has reduced our economic output, caused grocery stores to increase prices, put Americans out of work and has killed over 4,000 people in our country. No need for ballistic missiles here. Something invisible is among us, and it's lethal.

In the midst of all this is a constant stream of negativism coming from a liberal media and politicians who ride the coattails of journalistic bias. Criticism of the American President is a daily message coming from most T.V. and radio networks. Instead of praising health-care first responders, police and fire-safety workers, undermining of national efforts is taking place because of lingering hatred of the presidential candidate who was successful in 2016. Ah, Hell, let me relate what some Americans are doing to relieve the tension from staying at home.

Last evening on our patio, Madame et moi were enjoying different-colored liquids and maintaining social distancing when one of our building's residents approached carrying the drink of his choice. Our patio is big enough to accommodate four or five people and still mitigate…We asked our neighbor to join us. "But, weren't you supposed to stay inside?" Oh, shut up. Our neighbor had just gone through a severe back operation, and watching Gunsmoke 12 hours a day demands less mitigating. So, in our conversation with the neighbor, he shared something he thought appropriate to fit his own stay-at-home living situation. He told us that he had contacted his two daughters and their spouses by phone and suggested that they go out to dinner. Huh? One daughter lives in Arizona, the other in Indiana. He had sent them and their spouses enough money for a take-out dinner complete with wine of their choice. On a designated evening, by phone (skype) everyone would connect with one another and share a meal together. Oh, there was a catch. Each female guest was to wear their favorite dress, the men would wear suits. High-heeled shoes for the women, of course. I am eager to learn the result of this innovative outing. I'll keep you informed without mentioning my neighbor's name. You don't need to know everything!

In our New York community, our granddaughter, enamored with her sweetheart of two years is going through a similar mitigation…there's that word again. Both seniors in high school, my granddaughter sits on her front porch while her boyfriend sits in his truck in the driveway. They converse and discuss whether will begin after April 19, the day when classes are supposed to start after the recent shutdown. The lesson from all this? Simple. If a seventeen-year-old can follow rules about staying home, playground basketball players, adult pickle ball players and party animals could do the same. Just sayin'.

Pressures do not cease for those in political office. Just off the coast of Florida, not far from the port of Fort Lauderdale, floats a Holland America cruise ship. On board that ship are dozens of vacationers who are infected with a flu-like virus. Four people have died. Governor Ron DeSantis is now requesting that President Trump make a decision on whether the ship be allowed to dock. Uneasy rests the head who wears the crown. We do know, don't we, that no matter what decision the President makes, it will be wrong.

As indicated by both the President and his medical staff, the next two weeks will be crucial for Americans. In my case, a decision will have to be made. My wife and I are scheduled to fly out of Phoenix for Albany and then by car to Saratoga Springs. Will there be social distancing aboard the plane? Will planes be flying cross country to New York State? Flip a coin. Whether we mitigate here or there, we will remain strong. All of us.

In the last four days, 1,000 Americans per day have died from the virus. U.S. infections reached 216,000; deaths are at 5,100. World-wide figures are at 958, 000 confirmed cases and 47,208 deaths. The prognosis from scientists, physicians and world leaders is not promising, and we have been told that the worst is yet to come. Our economy as well as our health and wellbeing has also been affected. Labor statistics put 6.6 million out of work and applying for unemployment benefits. The Stock Market is at its lowest point in a decade. Should we go on? Damn right.

The State of Arizona announced this morning that the Grand Canyon Park, that enormous beautiful natural wonder is now closed until further notice. Major League Baseball opening has already been cancelled as has the Wimbledon Tennis Tournament. The latter was only cancelled twice in history—once in WWI and again in WWII. There will be no NCAA basketball finals this year. College football spring practice will not take place and whether the fall football season takes place or not has yet to be decided. In New York City, finally after too many weeks, playgrounds and basketball courts have been shut down.

At yesterday's White House Briefing, something new

took place. The Secretary of Defense, Mark Esper and his military chiefs of staff announced that drug interdiction would now be taking place at an increased rate. All branches of the military would be used to slow and impede the flow of drugs into the United States from South America. It was reported that the drug cartels have been using the lull in border crossings to increase traffic across the border. A fifty percent increase in interdiction efforts will now take place, and ships at sea as well as aircraft and ground forces will enhance the ability of United States anti-drug forces. One of the members of the Joint Chiefs of Staff reported that, "We are at war with COVID-19 and the drug cartels."

Some are united in this effort. Some are not. Yesterday's Boston Globe carried an editorial in which the President had "Blood on his hands." This reportedly was stated since the President was either not early enough in his initial response to the virus or wanted to put Americans back to work earlier. Adam Schiff in the House of Representatives is now looking into forming a committee to investigate the President's handling of the crisis. Here we go again! Talk about fiddling while the city burns! Oh, well.

Other Americans are being a little more positive. An outdoor birthday party was recently held for a 100-year-old female veteran. Social distancing was used and neighbors drove by in their cars to wish the centenarian happy birthday. In another community, a neighbor stands outside his home every morning with children standing next door, and they all recite the Pledge of Allegiance to the flag. Christmas lights are beginning to shine on several homes. Flags are being flown. Ah, but in my gated community, we, too, are making an effort to show pride in our unity. On our site, there are several three-story buildings housing permanent and part-time residents. On our side of the building, we have outdoor patios which look out onto the little roadway which separates buildings. On Saturday, April 4 at 5 P.M., four of us, two with banjos, one with a keyboard, a ninety-two-year-old church pianist, and one with a guitar will play, one-after-the-other, their special songs. So, from four patios, two on the second floor, two on the ground floor, we will have a party. No, Elton John will not host the event. We have asked that 6' to 10' distancing be adhered to by those wishing to listen. Will we have a folding-chair audience? Who knows? Let me get back to you. In the meantime, shelter-in-place, socially distance yourself, and remain on the firing line. Sticking together in this fight will at least make us feel good.

Let's go back a day or two. Do you remember my neighbor's idea of having dinner with his two daughters and their spouses via an Internet hookup? Here's some feedback. Speaking with him last evening, news of the dinner party proved interesting. Each branch, my neighbor and his wife and the two daughters and their spouses, used laptop computers. In full dinner dress, while having the meal, many miles apart, the groups enjoyed food, beverages and conversations which cemented in a family outing. The feeling of having come together, but yet separated by distance, was so fulfilling that another session is now being planned. One of my neighbor's daughters will select the next theme. I'll keep you posted. Now, back to reality, and it's not good.

Turmoil in the workplace, perhaps brought on from the stress of not knowing the exact procedures to follow when in crisis mode, has led to some concern. Health-care providers are now protesting outside hospitals because they feel that enough is not being done to provide them with protective materials—masks, gowns and face shields. In Guam, the Commander of the USS Theodore Roosevelt, one of America's aircraft carriers, was relieved of command because he alerted too many people including some overzealous journalists who leaked the fact that many of the ship's crew were ill with the 19 virus. To add to all this misery, over seven hundred thousand American workers are now unemployed, and a 4.4% unemployment level has been reached. That number is expected to reach 10% of the workforce.

China has once again come under scrutiny. 3M Company has been accused of making face masks in China and selling them to countries other than the United States. It is alleged that China has ordered that anything made in China stays in China. President Trump is now thinking of evoking the War Powers Act in order to have an American company comply with America's needs. This argument adds emphasis to the fact that American business, especially the pharmaceutical industry, return to American shores. Is there any good news? Some.

Celebrities such as Leonardo DiCaprio, Dolly Parton, Taylor Swift and others have contributed money to food programs and have offered monetary assistance intended to keep people in their jobs. The Boston Patriots' Team Plane was sent to China and returned with a load of badly-needed face masks. Ah, but there are some who constantly preach a doom and gloom dogma. Governor Cuomo often says that the United States will never be the same. He might be right, but the American people need a ray of hope. They need to know that the same stuff which made this Nation great is still running through the blood of its people. Yes, we should be cautious. We should adhere to social distancing, and if we have masks, we should wear them. But, if we are to win this war against an unseen enemy, we must remain together while we stay apart. Today's counts of those who tested positive and who died?

World-wide totals for contagion are at 1,000,000. Deaths are at 51,485. In the United States, those testing positive for the disease are at 245,500. Six thousand Americans have died so far.

APRIL 4, 2020

If I did not start today's commentary with a dialog on masks, an opportunity to showcase American or human ingenuity would be lost. Governors, medical personnel, our Nation's best scientists and health-care first responders are now in tizzy over the lack of N-95 masks, a simple cloth respirator manufactured by 3M and other companies. The American President has recently criticized 3M for making and sending such masks to Canada and other nations. Heated arguments have ensued over the dwindling supply of these simple life savers. That is just nuts! Look in your drawers and pull out a pair of undershorts or panties. There, right before your eyes are pairs of washable, ready-to-wear N-95 masks. A simple video, found online, shows how such undergarments can be fitted tightly and safely over your mouth, nose and ears. Good God, a simple adjustment of clothing we have in our homes does the job. Put your scissors, needles and plastic away and start wearing your Calvin Kleins, and bring down the cost of paper masks. I suggest using something not worn in the last few days.

Now, let's get back to the battle against this thing which is tearing us apart physically, mentally and economically. Contagion across the world is increasing. Today's counts world-wide are at 1.1 million confirmed cases. Deaths are at 60,000. In the U.S., confirmed cases are at 278, 550 while deaths are at 7,200. American deaths from 19 are still going up at a rate of 1,000 per day. Americans infected are mounting at a rate of 30,000 a day. Both figures are alarming. So are visits to the grocery stores.

Yesterday, in what I hope is one of my last visits for two weeks, empty shelves for paper goods still remind us of either hoarding or depleting stock piles of essential goods. Markers, signs, footprints painted on the floors remind us to adhere to social distancing. Plastic shields separate us from gloved checkout clerks who wear masks designed for health-care workers. Put your panties on! Fellow shoppers eye you with suspicion; *Are you an asymptomatic person?* Other supermarket personnel are wiping down shopping carts as if they were car-wash employees. Americans had become used to seeing a cornucopia of food items on display. Not anymore! Oh, yeah, masked fellow shoppers make the entire experience Mardi-Gras like. Eerie! Depressing? Certainly. We need someone to step and give a Billy Graham-type positive message…don't we.

Countries across the globe are now closing their borders, perhaps too late, but the concept of open borders has left the building. Focus is now being placed on saving the lives of those who are, oops, legal residents. What a concept! Other things are being shut down, too. Disney World, national parks, historic sites and public swimming pools are off limits. Sheltering-in-place is easier if there is no place to go. And, our education and our use of words is changing.

More than several seldom-used expressions are now common place. SARS-Cov-2 is one of these. Any new virus causing respiratory problems is so designated. We already are familiar with shelter-in-place and social distancing. Epicenter, that area with the highest counts of contagion is with us. Mitigation, the preparations that one can make to mitigate or lessen the impact of the disease has come up. The asymptomatic person, that individual who can transmit the virus as though a stealth bomber, is among us. The word, immunocompromised is used to define a weakened or impaired immune system. Hey, I am not a medical doctor. But I still avoid touching my face, and yes, I'm breaking out my Calvin Kleins.

Will humans continue to test positive and die from the virus in the coming days? Probably along with the Sun rising in the east. Will new ways to mitigate the effects of this thing take place? Hell, yes. We are Americans, and most of us are on the front lines.

APRIL 5, 2020

On this day, the news from medical and government officials is dire. White House members of the anti-Coronavirus Response Team report that this week will be the toughest for Americans. The President stated that, "There will be a lot of deaths." O19vernight records seem to reinforce that warning. World counts of those infected reached 1,203, 099, an increase of 100 thousand. World-wide deaths reached 64,774, an increase of almost 5,000 overnight. U.S. figures are not much better. Americans who tested positive number 312,245, an increase of 30,000 overnight. U.S. deaths from the virus reached 8,503, a jump of over 1,000 from yesterday. And, we are now told that the week ahead of us will be worse. Such news on Palm Sunday seems inappropriate and completely out of place.

Medical and scientific officials are comparing the Spanish flu of 1917 with the COVID-19. Over one hundred years ago, 100 million people died over the world. Will those figures be repeated or even surpassed? Some of us will soon find out. In the midst of all this doom and gloom, the President hinted that professional sports and attendance at such events might return to normal as soon as September.

Will the warmer summer months help stem the virus and help us return to normal? We will see. Let me get personal.

My permanent residence is in upstate New York, the State with the largest number of infected people. Today, there are 122,033 confirmed cases of 19. New York City is hard pressed to provide care for its population. Supplies, for one reason or another, are lacking. Planning, logistics and lack of oversight might be questioned. Governor Cuomo holds a daily briefing concerning efforts to help his state. Politics sometimes creep in his daily comments, family members often play a role in his description of how residents are coping, but he does outline some of the basic fears we are experiencing. This morning, cabin fever was discussed. This isolation has caused mood swings, irrational outbursts and has disturbed the domestic tranquility of many Americans. To add injury to insult, hundreds of New York State prisoners have been released who were contaminated with the virus. Such a burden should not have been added to the weight most residents are carrying.

On April 22, Madame et moi will fly out of Phoenix on our way to upstate New York. What might we encounter along the way, and how will we cope once there? At our age, eighty plus, we have some reservations. That, however, might make for an interesting documentation. The waiting in line for boarding, the flight among others crowded into cramped quarters, deplaning for transfers and final arrival into a state with the highest number of infected Americans—all this will or will not be recorded. We shall see. Now, let's have some fun and look at how some Arizona residents spent last evening.

A week ago, one of my fellow condo dwellers suggested

that we, two banjo players and one guitarist/vocalist, get together and hold a small musical salute to America from our patios in our community. We entitled the event as the "1ˢᵗ Annual Building 25 'From the Patios' Social Distancing Curb-Side Musical Salute to America." A flyer was posted in the building's elevator, and two banjo players and one guitarist practiced. Last evening, beginning at 5 P.M., the three of us (yes, I plunk along in a very amateur way) positioned ourselves on the ground level a half hour before we were to begin our "not-for-prime-time" presentation. To our surprise, over forty people showed up with folding chairs and positioned themselves along the narrow thoroughfare separating buildings. Various masks were worn, and that added *couleur locale* to the festivities. Not only did our audience listen, they applauded after every one-after-the-other song, and although they kept their social distancing, neighbors seemed to feel comfortable together. But, at the end, one of my fellow musicians ended the mini concert with his rendition of "America". It was a perfect ending, and after a genuine acknowledgement of appreciation, most people uttered, "God bless America." Good thing CNN was not there. 'God' just doesn't seem to fit in on their coverage. I wish I had performed as well as my fellow players. Oh, well. Perfect practice makes perfect.

Oh, one more thing…sorry. At the end of the mini concert, the community's social director asked the stringed instrument players if they could do a similar show on a monthly basis. That ain't gonna happen.

APRIL 6, 2020

The Surgeon General of the United States says that this week will be "our Pearl Harbor moment." President Trump tells us that this will be "the toughest week yet." Most Americans have been advised to shelter-at-home, use social distancing and to wear a mask if the need arises to go outside, to the supermarket or to the pharmacy. One of the White House specialists, Dr. Fauci, suggests that the entire country should be in lockdown. That idea was quickly disputed by one of Wyoming's United State Senators who said that people in his state are already separated by miles from each other on ranches, farms and rural communities. Not so in upstate New York.

In a call from our daughter in Saratoga Springs yesterday, my wife and I were told that she had received a phone call from county officials stating than anyone going to the grocery store, pharmacy or gas station, would be required to wear a mask. New York State is battening down the hatches in the face of rising numbers of contagion and death from the virus. Today's counts world-wide for 19 are at 1,288,474 confirmed cases. Deaths are at 70,569. In the United States, there are 336,907 confirmed cases and 9,624 deaths. In less than twenty-four hours, the United States will surpass more than 10,000 who will have died from the virus.

Most Americans are conforming to requirements about staying at home. There are still cyclists, walkers on the streets and bike paths, but the number of exercise seekers is dwindling. How the contagion is spread is still not clear to even the specialists governing the virus. This morning, it was learned that the Bronx Zoo just reported that one of its tigers, a four-year old big cat had contracted the virus from one of its handlers who did not know that he was infected. Other big cats have symptoms of the disease. Big cats becoming infected? Brings something to mind. Americans love their animals. Almost 3 out of 5 Americans (I am not sure of the percentage. Ask the CEO of Microsoft. He's good with numbers.) So, animal lovers. Be careful when you walk your pets. They don't wear shoes, and they track almost anything back into the home. Might not want to kiss them too much. I know that I am not going close to my tiger.

So, how is 19 contracted? Scientists tell us to wash our hands as often as possible and not to touch our face. Wearing a mask, whether it is made from a pair of Calvin Kleins or a D-cup bra, is a good idea. Can the thing, this god-awful pandemic, come through window panes, slink down chimneys, slip under front doors, and drop down on you from trees like Florida iguanas in cold weather? Remains to be seen once the guys with the microscopes discover what it is. Is hiding under your desk as was advocated in the 1950's helpful? Probably not. But it does seem that the best idea so far is hunkering down at home…with the dog and cat. I wonder if the wine store clerk will let me in when I come through the front door wearing my colorful mask.

Many Americans are concerned about the economy. Those out of work will get a temporary reprieve once they receive funds from the 2.2 trillion dollar Relief Package. However, most of those funds will last for one month. The President, his administration and the country had enjoyed an unprecedented booming economy. Will the effects of virus be abated enough to all a back-to-work ethic? We will perhaps be better informed at the end of this week. It will be a tough one. Even world leaders are not immune from 19. Boris Johnson, the U.K. Prime Minister is now in hospital with the disease. The spouse of Canada's Prime Minister has fallen ill with the virus. So, in this cataclysmic week, curb your cabin fever and ride it out. I'm still concerned about the wine-clerk's reaction. Will he or she be armed?

APRIL 7, 2020

Here we are in the second day of what is supposed to be the toughest week of our battle against 19, this ugly, contagious virus from who knows where. We were alerted yesterday that even animals can be infected from contact with humans. Not a good sign. However, it was reported that, for the first time, fewer people in New York City tested positive for the virus. In the United States, reports do not support a decline. Americans who contracted the disease are not at 368,241. Deaths are at 10,986, still more than one thousand per day. World-wide figures of confirmed rest at 1,347, 892, and deaths at 74,808. Whether we have reached the apex in this increasing contagion is unsure. One thing is sure. Americans in future decades will remember what has taken place these last few months, and along with the Spanish flu of 1917, they will remember COVID-19 along with Pearl Harbor and 9/11.

New York's Governor Cuomo has doubled the fine of not adhering to shelter-in-place directives to $1,000, and he has closed the schools until April 29. In other news, the Prime Minister of the U.K., Boris Johnson, is now in the Intensive Care Unit in London. In the United States and across the globe, domestic violence has increased. Cabin fever is seemingly taking its toll in homes where people are cooped up for long periods of time. Tension, patience and tolerance are tested daily by this unseen enemy, and that same antipathy has played a role in how many Americans view the 45th President of the United States.

My first sighting and recognition of Donald J. Trump came in the mid 1990's. While visiting my son who was working in Brooklyn at the time, we decided to attend a Marine Corps birthday celebration taking place at a Manhattan restaurant/bar, 'Liquid Assets' in the Wall Street area. At the same time, people were lining the streets waiting for the St. Patrick's Day Parade to take place. We decided to watch the procession as it passed by. Two of the marchers were Donald Trump and his then wife, Marla Maples. My son and I agreed that the businessman and his wife made a striking couple. When the marriage broke up in 1999, I wondered how a man could leave such a beautiful woman and his daughter. It is easy to judge others from a distance.

After the divorce, and before he met and married Melania, the present 1st Lady, the Donald was rumored to have had dalliances with other young women. Boys will be boys…won't they. Then, early in the first decade of the 21st century, in 2004, Trump hosted a T.V. show entitled, 'The Apprentice'. In that popular program, Trump showed himself to be crass, caustic, stern and abrasive. Negative image? Not really. Many Americans grew tolerant of a man who demanded excellence of his staff, and when he would say at the end of each show, "You're fired!", some of the audience liked a person who expected competence of his staff. About the same time, the 44th President of the United States was apologizing to the world claiming that his country had been arrogant and that America was never exceptional. Americans do not like to be told that they are second in anything. Along came the presidential election of 2016.

The Democrat contender for the presidency was Hillary Clinton, a former 1st Lady, Senator, and Secretary of State. Loved by a liberal media, the darling of House of Representative members, Clinton carried some heavy baggage. Just before her nomination for candidacy, the Secretary had been seen as not providing security and safety to Embassy personnel in Benghazi, the scene of a military and diplomatic debacle. Enter Donald Trump, a non-politician, an outsider.

In a contested election, Trump was elected President. But, from the moment of his nomination and into the first months of his presidency, Trump came under fire from all sides of the aisle.

One thing after another was brought up disputing the Trump Presidency. First, he was accused by Obama appointees of the FBI for having colluded with Russia and the Ukraine. In what appeared to be a complete political bias on the part of FBI officials, all charges of collusion were tabled. However, an immediate uproar from Democrats in the House of Representatives, headed up by Adam Schiff, Nancy Pelosi, Maxine Waters and others, a move to impeach the President ensued. For more than three months, the very time when elected officials should have been focused on a disease which was ravaging China, the House of Representatives impeached the President. In the end, the President was exonerated of all charges. People began to like Donald J. Trump.

Where to begin. Things are happening and falling like dominoes in a windstorm. Yesterday, the Secretary of the Navy, Thomas Modly, resigned after receiving criticism for his having removed the captain of the USS Theodore Roosevelt aircraft carrier and calling the captain "stupid" for his asking for help from higher ups in letters. One of those letters was intercepted by a journalist seeking attention and leaked to the public. The captain of the aircraft carrier was removed from command, and he will probably retire quietly and play golf in some shoreline community. Boris Johnson, the Prime Minister of the U.K. is in hospital in the I.C. unit recovering from contracting the virus. The city of New York is going through its toughest week in confirmed cases of the disease, but Governor Cuomo reports that an apex might have been reached. However, across the country, the deadly disease is gaining ground.

Hot beds of infection are now rising up in Chicago, New Orleans and other metropolitan areas. The African-American Mayor of Chicago reported that more African-Americans are dying from the disease than any other ethnic group. In response to that claim, Dr. Ben Carson, Director of Housing and Urban Development, explained that many African-Americans suffer from diabetes, obesity, asthma, and hypertension, health problems which lead to susceptibility to death from contracting 19. In what is disturbing, New York and Louisiana saw the highest deaths in one day.

World-wide statistics on the disease show 1,431,375 confirmed cases, an increase of almost 100,000 in one day. World-wide deaths are at 82,145, over 7,000 in one day. In the United States, 399,886 confirmed cases are recorded, over a 30,000 increase from yesterday. U.S. deaths are at 12, 907. Spain has 14,045 dead, Italy is at 17,127, France has 10,343, Germany at 2,016 (do German people really follow orders?). But, an extraordinary figure of recorded deaths comes from China which puts its total of deaths at only 3,337. For the second highest population of any nation on Earth, for a starting off point of the disease, that figure is now disputed by almost everyone including the American President. In an announcement yesterday, President Trump suggested that funding to the World Health Organization be stopped. WHO has cozied up to China in its disclosures of numbers reported and it has backed China's hesitancy to share other information related to the disease. Frustration over the lack of solid information on the disease is taking place on the home front.

Domestic violence, perhaps from being cooped up, social distancing and sheltering-in-place, has increased. People are eating more, exercising less, and resorting to alcohol and drugs, not a good recipe for good mental and physical health. In spite of that fact, Dr. Anthony Fauci and others have announced that Americans might see a turnaround by the end of this week if mitigation is adhered to as advised.

In other news, Governor Cuomo has extended his no school advisory through April 29, and he has doubled the fine of not using social distancing to $1,000. Another 250 billion dollars is being asked from Congress to help bolster the economy. Questions are now being asked whether the warmer spring and summer's heat might eradicate or lessen the spread of the disease. That question might have come about because Americans want to return to what might never be a normal life. We will find out…together.

APRIL 9, 2020

At this, our toughest week in the fight against 19, the Nation is faced with 6.6 million jobless claims. One of the Democrat contenders for the presidency, Bernie Sanders, has dropped out of the race but insists that his quest to bring his socialist agenda to the Democrat's Convention will continue. In New York State, the governor tells us that "We are flattening the curve." Social distancing, a mitigation daily advised by medical personnel, seems to be working. And there are several findings which indicate a possible social change that will come about because of the virus.

Medical doctors are now stating that smokers are more vulnerable to testing positive for COVID-19 since the disease is respiratory. Damage to the lungs due to tobacco and electronic derivatives (vaping) makes it easier for the virus to enter the body and do harm. Will such information cause smokers to be more cautious? Maybe. But statistics show that smokers are three times more prone to be affected by the virus than non-smokers. Thousands of airplanes are now parked on tarmacs, and some of them, because of lack of constant maintenance, will never fly again. In place of flying back and forth across the United States to visit family and friends, Americans and others throughout the world are using electronic hookups. That aspect of socialization will be discussed later in this chapter.

Are world and national numbers of contagion and death going up? Today's world-wide positive cases are at 1,484,810, up 80 thousand over yesterday. World-wide deaths stand at 88,538, 6 thousand over 24 hours. Americans with the disease are at 432,132, 30 thousand over yesterday. Two thousand more Americans died and that figure is at 14,817. We are still in what has been termed as the worst week of the war against the beast. In spite of the bad news, there are those who are calling for a date when Americans can get back to work. But, now, in the fog of this war, let's take a look at what might really be important.

Think back to a couple days ago when I mentioned that my neighbor had collaborated with his two daughters and their spouses and a dinner party was held online. That effort, perhaps inspired by the virus, its unknowns, its lethality and the belief that family connections are important, made me reflect on my own family. Within the past several days, my wife and I have talked to our children, a man and a woman who live in Texas and in upstate New York, almost daily. Hum! And, why not? The 'kids' are good ones. We refer to them as 'our favorite son' and 'our favorite daughter'. Let me tell you about them. Oh, shut up. I'm writing here!

Our first-born, Brooks Marcel, was conceived in Quebec when I was a student at Université Laval. We have always maintained that he is Canadian-American, and he speaks French well enough to qualify. Growing up, Brooks' father loved him, but due diligence did not give me the time to appreciate that little boy. Later, after trying college, he joined the United States Marine Corps much to the chagrin of his mother. However, as a Marine, he was more outstanding than his father in the sense that he was paint-your-face, rubber-boat, go-out-at night warrior. He is now a recipient of a wounded-veteran supplement, and he made sure the government put him through four years of university study at Campbell University in North Carolina. He married a wonderful girl/woman from Puerto Rico, a multilingual business woman who tolerates her stay-at-home husband who prepares the meals, does the household chores, takes care of our three grandchildren, their dog and still has time to do the laundry and ride his motorcycle with Dick Armey, a former Congressman from Texas. Brooks' mother and father love him and his family.

My favorite daughter? Janine Michelle grew into a sensational young woman. In high school, she was an athlete. She was the best catcher on her softball team, a basketball player and a super volleyball player. In undergraduate school, she played rugby. Her college major was elementary education, and she was destined to be a teacher. However, I jokingly tell Janine that she majored in sorority, an organization which took too much of her study time. And, I even had a sweatshirt made up for her which read, "Alpha Humpta Dumpta". At Plattsburgh University in New York State, she graduated, but instead, married her high school sweetheart and raised two children. That's when things turned for the better and our 'favorite daughter' found her calling in life.

As a young woman, Janine returned to Plattsburgh and earned her master's degree in elementary education, and she graduated with honors. Knowing that she wanted to spend time with her own children, Janine started a child-care business serving only children of teachers in the area which gave her the same free time as had her own children. Children under her care often invite Janine to high school graduation ceremonies later in life and cite her as having influenced them in their formative years. She still worked actively in her profession right up until the closing of school which Governor Cuomo is keeping closed until April 29 or longer if necessary. Besides being highly sought after as a day-care operator, Janine has made a name for herself as one of the area's best Zumba instructors. Janine's mother and father love her and her family.

What did you expect? In these times, things should be said to those you love. Do it often, and if you get a chance to write about them in a chronicle, don't worry about what some readers, some literary critics or some book publishers say. What the Hell do they know about life? I think I'll make a call or two.

OK, is it getting any better? It depends on where you are. If you are in the New York City area, there have been over 7,000 deaths from 19. However, it has been reported that fewer people are being admitted to hospital. If you look at world-wide and U.S. statistics, a more realistic opinion takes place. Throughout the world, 1,617,204 confirmed cases are reported with 97,039 deaths. Both figures show increases over twenty-four hours. In the United States, 466,299 confirmed cases are followed with 16,886 deaths. Over 2,000 deaths compared to yesterday's counts. As predicted, this is our worst week yet. On the political and informational stage, criticism is still rampant.

James Carville, a political aide-de-camp of Bill Clinton, just quipped, "The GOP will kill people to stay in power." Pretty strong accusation, James. The media is now attacking President Trump over his handling of the crisis facing us. They must have the answers, but no one seems to be able to put a definite brake on the swift-moving pandemic. A U.S. Senator from Texas says that the only way to defeat the virus is to get the American economy running again. Models of what could be the apex of both deaths and contagion are proving to be wrong, and that leaves doubt in everyone's mind. A new formula, that of the R/o or R naught, relating to the rate of infection from those who have tested positive is on the books. Anyone understand all this? Please step up if you do. Even the World Health Organization has come under scrutiny.

President Trump recently questioned the WHO for having received millions of dollars from the United States and then backing Chinese claims of few fatalities after paying the health organization less than 20% of what Americans had paid. One T.V. talking head from Fox News said, "China lied, the world died" in suggesting that China did not disclose the truth of the disease's breakout last December. And, on the home front, politics is again playing havoc with efforts to relieve economic stress on Americans.

The Senate has proposed a bill to extend a large amount of money to small businesses which could collapse without it. The House of Representatives has stated that more money is needed for women and people of color to bolster their businesses before any additional funding is voted in. The inability to agree that there are Americans already trying to pay their workers while not doing business is not helping our nation move past this crisis. Perhaps the present religious season will help relieve the tension.

Today is Good Friday, two days before Easter. The Jewish Passover took place Wednesday. However, churches remain empty. Large-group congregations are frowned upon, and religious services will be held electronically across the world. Will the feeling of togetherness while miles apart creep into the human psyche? Let's hope so. 19's big scythe is cutting a wide swath through us. Time to dull the blade.

Well, here we are. We have reached the end of what was reported to be the toughest week of the siege. Let's check statistics. In New York State, the hardest hit of all fifty, 174, 489 confirmed cases of the virus have been recorded. Seven thousand, eight-hundred and eighty-seven deaths have taken place. The number of people testing positive has stayed relatively flat. While the NY daily death toll is staggering, 777 deaths in one day, the rate of coronavirus patients in hospital has shown signs of dropping. Officials had estimated that 140,000 hospital beds might be needed, only about 18,500 were in use by week's end. Good news. But this scourge is still lurking close by.

World-wide totals of contagion and death continue to rise. Those testing positive are at 1,698, 626. Deaths are at 102,774, an additional 5,000 over yesterday's figures. In the United States, those contracting the disease are at 501,560. American deaths are at 18,777, two thousand more than yesterday. And, the battle continues to rage. On the home front, other things, both good and bad are taking place.

The President wants May 1 to be the day for reopening the country. He repeatedly says, "This country was made to be open." Trump has said that reopening the American economy will be the biggest decision of his life. He may be right. Past predictions that up to 2.2 million lives could be lost seem to be false. One task-force member stated that Americans could be back to normal by November. That same individual cautions us that social distancing has brought about a change in projections and that the mitigation of the virus must be continued. Probably so. But people are getting bored. One can watch reruns of T.V. sitcoms for only so long. Libraries, gyms, restaurants, parks, playgrounds, swimming pools and beaches and nightclubs remain dormant. Social distancing has exasperated the situation, and in-home relations can become strained. Efforts to further help those out of work are now being hindered by partisan politics.

The Senate has proposed another aid program for out-of-work Americans. The House majority is dragging its feet because they want more money for family planning, minority and women's work programs and additional funding for PBS, things which do not pertain to the problem at hand. However, the most problematic proposal by House members Adam Schiff and Carmella Harris is the suggestion that a House Investigative Committee begin a 9/11-type probe of the handling of the Coronavirus outbreak. Will we see another three to four-month long inquiry into the efforts of Donald J. Trump? Sure looks like it. And, the hatred of the American President does not stop in the halls of Congress.

Recently, the White House press staff balked at a One America News reporter being offered a chair at the WH Briefing Room. Finally, the press corps asked that the pro-administration young reporter be placed standing at the back of the room. In her place, on separate days, two Chinese reporters, one of whom suggested that China was ready to help in any way it could, were offered the OAN reporter's chair. Bias, hatred, partisan, evil, childlike? Your pick.

Tomorrow is Easter Sunday. Many if not all churches will be empty. However, religious services will take place on T.V. networks and on radio. Some well-known evangelists will conduct services and bring messages of hope to millions of Americans at home and abroad. Robert Jeffress will be with President Trump in a lap-top hookup on this religious date. They will share messages of peace and strength together will we watch. Will those messages help soothe the pain and frustration many are feeling? Hopefully.

Happy Easter!

Let's get right to it. The U.S. death toll from the 19 virus now tops Italy's for the highest in the world. Twenty thousand and six-hundred and eight Americans have died from the disease. Two thousand more Americans died over the last twenty-four hours from the contagion, and total Americans testing positive is 529, 951, up 28,000 from yesterday. World-wide figures for those testing positive are at 1,777,666, and by tomorrow, those figures will close in on two million infections world-wide. Deaths across the globe rest at 108,867, up six thousand since yesterday.

In other news related to the virus, the President has declared every state in the Union to be eligible for Federal Disaster Designation. Apple and Google have alerted I-phone users that an app is now available which will alert phone users to determine whether they have come in contact with someone infected with COVID-19. In what is no surprise, the somewhat tainted New York Times has declared that President Trump knew about the virus before it struck. Hum? In Texas, the Court of Appeals has upheld the state's decision to curtail abortions for another month citing that surgeons are needed in the fight against the virus and should be made available for other operations. Real Estate agents are now showing available housing via virtual open houses. The President is considering opening the American economy by the end of May. But Americans are still concerned, and they are talking while observing social distancing.

So, a few of us brave souls were talking on our patio last night. Oh, yes, socially distanced and sheltered-in-place, of course, and discussing T.V. shows. "Did you see, 'Bosch'?" "Yes, for the 17th time, all six seasons!" "How about, 'Justified'?" "Yes, that, too." And, on it went. One person, a real talker, repeated for the 27th time in two days, "I'm bored." We just nodded in agreement. Sound like your own cautious but every-day discussion? The libraries and closed. The gyms, parks, playgrounds, bars, restaurants, shops, hair and nail salons and movies are closed. Grocery stores are open, but everybody looks like Bonnie and Clyde, and if you approach a bank to do business, there are John Dillinger look-alikes all over the place. The masks people are wearing are more colorful than spring flowers. On my daily bike ride on my one-speed, coaster-brake antique, I keep thinking that I am under attack by masked bandits. But the masked riders usually nod or say hello as they speed by. Even in this time of a silent, invisible, lethal killer, some people even say, "Happy Easter."

My distaste for American politics is at its apex. Now, there's a word. New York Times tells us daily that the President could have acted earlier in closing down the nation. Hum? Wasn't he being impeached by the House of Representatives at the time? Shouldn't the entire government have been watching events in China concerning a silent, more lethal virus than the flu? Oh, well. CNN has echoed the Times claim, and even Dr. Fauci, a member of the President's Task Force against the virus has stated that sheltering-in-place should have taken place earlier. It is hard to disagree with such a view. However, if we would have closed our borders in November last year…You know the rest. Instead of going back and using supposition, we should move forward and fight the disease.

More face masks are seen everywhere. And, for the most part, Americans are adhering to social distancing. But, as one Marine high up in the riggings of one of John Paul Jones' ships reacted to the order, "Don't give up the ship!", he said, "Ten percent never get the word." Who could have imagined that over 557, 663 Americans would have tested positive (today's figures) for a virus that no one can detect, isolate or cure? Twenty-two thousand, one hundred and sixteen

Americans have died so far. World-wide confirmations of the virus are at 1,863,406 and deaths number 115,225. New York City cases of confirmed testing positive now top 100,000. Americans are getting itchy for change.

The President is contemplating the opening of the country and getting people back to work. I am sure he knows that whatever his decision, it will be termed wrong by those who hate the man, his family and his political affiliation. Trump has already stated that the decision to jump-start the economy will be the biggest decision he has ever made. Let's hope he makes the right decision.

Yesterday, Easter Sunday, several churches in Kansas and in other states held open religious services in spite of orders to remain in place. Frustration causes us to make spur of the moment decisions. The President knows that, too. Knowing that last week was supposedly the toughest week in our battle with the beast, let's see what today and tomorrow brings. Oh, this morning, a minor adjustment was made in the way we bring food into the home. A little before 6 A.M., I drove to the closest supermarket and found about eight to ten people standing in line, socially distanced by signs posted on the ground, waiting for the store to open. Promptly at 6, the doors opened and ten of us were allowed in. Number 11 had to wait until number 1 or his likeness exited the market. Get there early, get r' done, and get out.

In eight days, Madame et moi are scheduled to leave our winter home and return to upstate New York. We will perhaps take a flight out of Sky Harbor Airport via Southwest Airlines if indeed planes are still flying. Going to anywhere in the State of New York is not the most advisable thing to do at the moment, but things at our permanent residence need tending. And, there are certain advantages to taking that flight. If this chronicle is worth the effort, a recording of getting to an airport, checking in, boarding and transfers is important. Will fewer automobiles be on the roads leading up to the airport? Will we see hundreds of plans lined up on the tarmac? Will baggage handlers be masked, will social distancing be mandatory in check-in lanes and will the federal marshals be checking passports? What will the seating arrangements be like? Will we still be cramped and squeezed together like sardines? If the flight takes place and if our reservations are not cancelled, you will read more about all this in the April 22-23 entries. *Bon voyage?*

Where do I begin? Do we talk about the tornado devastation which took place in the American Southeast yesterday? Americans standing in awe looking at what used to be their homes and saddened by friends and neighbors who lost their lives in an act of God? Do I talk about late, not-yet received bailout payments enacted by the federal government weeks ago? Long lines at grocery stores, required face coverings, social distancing edicts, and worry about rent and mortgage payments face almost everyone. In the midst of all this is a bias and partisan media and political party which further divides and weakens a resolve to fight this plague.

In a comparison of yesterday's news, I watched CNN and other anti-Trump newscasts and compared them with One America News and Fox News. It was as if two separate stories were being told. The latter two reported on positive efforts the Trump Administration was making to relieve the tension and get America back to what has been termed, "the new normal". The former spoke of the President's efforts to rewrite history, i.e. make it appear that decisions made were faulty. Some things never change. But, statistics on the march of the virus did.

Twenty-three thousand, six hundred and forty-nine

Americans have died from the disease. Over 582,600 in the U.S. have been tested positive. World-wide, 1,930,780 tested positive and 120,450 have died. Over 1,000 Americans died yesterday. Throughout the world, over 5,000 more people succumbed to the disease. Yet, Washington is considering putting the U.S. back to work. While no specific date has yet been chosen for such a move, May 1 seems to be one target. The problem is a political divide; governors of individual states are now saying that they, not the President should decide. It will be interesting if a consensus can be reached.

Yesterday, in Guam, an American sailor who served aboard the USS Theodore Roosevelt, one of our aircraft carriers, succumbed to the disease. Over 500 other crew members tested positive to this fast-spreading contagion. It is suspected that while on liberty in Far Eastern ports, unsuspecting men and women picked up the virus. Not only is 19 taking toll of our economy and resolve, our military is now being weakened by an unseen enemy.

New York State's Governor Cuomo says that, "The worst is over." Could be. Doesn't seem like that. In France, the use of Chloroquine, the anti-malaria drug, is having positive results. Ninety-six percent of Frenchmen who have used the drug are virus-free after ten days. American medical professionals are perhaps overly cautious to promote its use. Ah, science. Isn't it wonderful!

Will we get back to work by the end of the month? Will Madame et moi be able to test our ability to get back to New York next week? *On verra.*

APRIL 15, 2020

For the last twenty-six days, world-wide and American numbers of positive cases and deaths from the virus have mounted. World-wide contagions have almost reached two million people at 1,999,628. Deaths across the globe are 128,601. Americans testing positive are at 609,685, and deaths are 26,059, up three thousand since yesterday. It is not over. Some experts claim that numbers are leveling off. Maybe.

Yesterday's news includes Barak Obama's endorsement of Joe Biden for president. That was expected. At the same time, America's former President campaigned against the incumbent president in what is perhaps an unprecedented move. Few if any past presidents ever say ill of those in office. Times have changed. Elsewhere, President Trump is threatening to withdraw funds from the World Health Organization for its close ties to China in the early moments of the breakout of the virus. The United States pays an enormous amount of money to WHO in comparison to China. Maybe some money can be saved here. However, again as expected, the President's move is being questioned by celebrities and the political opposition. Surprise, surprise!

In New York State, the death toll has reached 10,000.

In France, the famous *Tour de France* has been postponed. In Michigan, the public is protesting against Michigan's Governor saying that civil liberties are being threatened because of stay-at-home orders. Cabin fever is working its way into politics. School closing across America are disrupting the educational process, and parents as well as children are caught up in a new social change. But, the biggest call to arms remains the desire to get America back to work.

I wonder if our local, state and federal elected officials are aware of the American dilemma of gloom and despondency. Tornadoes have destroyed homes and taken lives throughout the Southeast. Unemployment is rampant across the country, and we are experiencing an economic downturn unseen since the Great Depression. Such things make some people wonder whether life is so important. Last evening on our AZ patio, yes, socially distanced, one man used one of his fingers, touched his nose and said, "There, I just committed suicide." OK, it was funny, and we needed some levity. But, elsewhere, for those who are not our age and not pensioned off, earning a living and providing for home and family are sources of worry and despair. Such thoughts should not be overlooked.

The only thing which might lessen the burden of staying-in-place might be getting America back to work. Now, what will it take to do that? Let's start with courage. Those going back to the workplace must know that, if they are afflicted with this disease facing all of us, they, the workers, will be taken care of…free of charge. Such people will jump start the economy. We must not allow partisan politics and a biased media to interfere. Hey my wife is eighty years old, she might…

Maybe not.

APRIL 16, 2020

Today's entry in this chronicle will be one of the last times reference is made to contagion and death throughout the world and in the United States. The end result and counts will be more relevant and perhaps provide hope. On March 19, the United States had 157 dead from the virus. Today, there are 30,985, and over 639,664 confirmed positive. A month ago, the world had 9,800 recorded deaths. Today, there are over 138,101 confirmed dead. Enough with the figures for contracting and dying from 19.

Instead of dwelling on the above, let's look at daily decision making throughout our world. This morning, Governor Cuomo in New York State declared that anyone in the streets, outdoors, etc. should wear a mask. While that edict was not mandatory, the governor emphasized the necessity of curbing the increase in infections. Medical professionals are now stating that contracting the disease may lead to lung and kidney diseases and that every part of the body could be affected. Not good news for anyone.

The Nation is still divided along political lines, and partisan bickering does hamper attempts to curb and defeat this enemy among us. The question of masks, whether to wear them or not, whether they thwart or enhance the march of this plague is still among us. Hospital personnel are still claiming that not enough PPE materials are provided, and there is a loud call for increased testing…in spite of the fact that developing such items takes time. Patience is in small supply along with needed materials. The call to go back to work is also pronounced, but states' rights is being used to slow any work starting. May 1 has been used as a date for back-to-work efforts, but, that, too, is a political football which bounces back and forth across the field of decision.

Been to stores other than the supermarkets lately? Yesterday, my computer was acting up, and I decided that a trip to Best Buy or Staples was necessary. Huh? Empty parking lots at the mall was the first sign that things had changed. Yellow police tape cordoned off areas where pickups only, with masked store personnel would deliver items ordered to your car, would take place. No one was allowed to enter the big-box Best Buy. Ah, but Staples was open. With my mask in place, I entered.

At the door, I was greeted by a masked something or other. I couldn't tell whether it was human or robot, male or female. I think it said, "May I burp you?" Perhaps it was, "May I help you?", but its mask got tied up with its tongue. After a short time, I decided that I would return to my prison of a home and try my luck with over-the-phone ordering. Our stores are now something right out of **1984.**

Let me wax personal a bit. So, here I am, in the declining moments of my life, reflecting back over things past. A lot of treasured memories come to mind. Living in a tar-paper shack, playing high school football with good friends, serving in the Marine Corps with those same friends, marrying the girl of my dreams and having two wonderful children. All those thoughts fly by quickly because my mind is occupied with the reality of the present—the threat of this terrible scourge ripping through the world. But, when one gives it serious thought, this 19 thing has brought some of us together. Americans seem less prone to find fault with one another. Family ties appear to be stronger than ever. People everywhere are communicating in better ways and with more sincerity. Sons, daughters, relatives and close friends are reaching out electronically in hookups in this shelter-in-place atmosphere.

In the federal government, elected officials, some, not all (partisan politics still raises its ugly head) are willingly accepting the challenge of trying to get Americans back to work, back to the future, i.e. the American way of life—the pursuit of happiness. So, in spite of being in the winter of my years, I look on with pride at Americans who just lost their homes and loved ones from the tornadoes which ravaged the Southeast, at those wage-earning hard-working people who lost their jobs, and yet, refuse to wave any white flag of surrender. Hell, these people still laughingly touch their nose with a finger and say, "There, take that you damned virus!" Admirable!

All sorts of news. In New York State, Governor Cuomo has extended the lockdown to May 15. Getting service in most stores other than the supermarket will be difficult. The wearing of masks when not sheltered-in-place is now mandatory in that state. In Washington, the President's Task Force against the virus has just announced a 3-Phase plan to reopen the economy. In phase 1, schools, bars, gyms and parks would remain closed. In phase 2, those same places would open but be subject to social distancing. In phase 3, a further relaxation of rules would take place and the economy would once again be active. All of the above is contingent upon avoiding a flare-up of the virus. We will be able to determine later whether or not the plan is or was successful.

The origin of the virus is still in question. However, American military and medical personnel point to a lab in the Chinese city of Wuhan as being the source of an experiment which, because of faulty work conditions, allowed the escape of the virus into the world. The World Health Organization has questioned this hypothesis, but the social distancing of this organization with China is in question.

In other more positive news, Boeing is rescheduled to begin production of airplanes in its plants. Certain members of Congress are considering a second relief package for American business. As one would expect, the Speaker of the House is requesting items not pertinent to the recovery of the economy be included in the bill. Ah, the inevitable ability of partisan politics to hold its sway.

And, the airlines! How could I not consider America's busiest transportation industry? Oops! Not anymore. Let's look at how 19 has affected our airlines. No more vapor trails in the sky. Clear blue skies overhead. We have already been told how Boeing, one of the largest aircraft builders in the world has been set back. Their problems began with newest member of their fleet, the 737 Max, was beset with mechanical difficulties. A few of those planes fell out of the sky and disrupted the entire manufacturing system. Fade to the present.

At the moment, thousands of airplanes are from all companies are parked on tarmacs throughout the Southwest. Dry weather slows the wear and tear on planes. Will these machines ever fly again? We have been told that airplane maintenance is geared to servicing planes which seldom are at rest. Those maintenance personnel are out of work as are the crews who fly the planes. Ah, but, let me get personal.

My wife and I were scheduled to depart from Phoenix, AZ and arrive in Albany, NY. Today, for the third time in one week, our flights were cancelled, and we had to rebook. Now, you say, "No big thing!" You think so? During all this turmoil, changes had to be made. T.V., phone, Wi-Fi and automobile insurances had to be adjusted in both states.

Transfers to and from airports had to be rescheduled. Was that all? Oh, Hell, no.

When one is leaving from one place to another, the United State Postal Service must be contacted and mail delivery changed. Hum? Who picks up your mail at your new destination if you are not there? Shutting down housekeeping in the old, and taking care of the new is sometimes a problem. Perishable food must be disposed of, household furniture must be cleaned and stored away. Enough? Nope. Early this morning, a fourth chance was announced via the Internet. We were counseled that we could cancel our reservations…and do all the requests for changes all over again. If and when we do take off, you will be made aware of what one encounters at the TSA, airport, checking in, boarding and flying with who knows how many others.

Overlooked was the closing of churches in response to social distancing. Weddings, planned a year earlier, had to be postponed, and when it is all said and done, some of those weddings will never take place. Sometimes, the spontaneous leads to longevity. When the opportunity is somehow taken away, relationships dissolve. Let's hope not.

Here we go again. In Washington, it has been decided, along with governors from each state, that an individual approach to opening America will be adhered to, and that trends in contagion will determine whether America gets back to work. In Florida, certain beaches are now open but for only eight hours per day. Gun shops in New Mexico are defying orders to remain closed, and owners of these stores say that they can control the six-foot mitigation laws. A second relief package designed to keep small businesses in operation is being held up in Congress. Once again, partisan politics has held up badly-needed funds to keep some businesses from going broke.

Elsewhere, the media is divided as to claims that China was at fault in either releasing or keeping secrets about the breakout of the COVID-19 pandemic. In Washington, it is reported that an experiment on bats infected with the virus went terribly wrong and the disease escaped a Chinese lab and worked its way into the wet markets of the city of Wuhan. Many in the United States are calling for an investigation into the incident, and a call for China to be held accountable is being loudly spread throughout the world. Will such an investigation ever take place? Perhaps.

However, the real secret, the actual truth of the matter will probably never be uncovered. Politics, diplomacy and caution will prevent that.

In further developments, it has been reported that truck drivers, so important in moving goods and services to the American public are in short supply. I wonder why. At the moment, my brother-in-law is a driver for the Dave Matthews Band. That entertainment group and hundreds of others across the United States is not on stage or not on tour. Each musical organization employs a half-dozen drivers of 18 wheelers which haul instruments, furniture, sets, lighting, etc. Those drivers are now out of work, and they are looking for employment. We are not short of truck drivers. It is just that the wrong people are looking in the wrong place.

At this juncture in the chronicle, it would be a serious oversight if I did not bring up another aspect of sheltering-in-place and socially distancing. It has already been mentioned that because of the above two mitigating circumstances, we could see a new crop of babies in the month of December. Divorces could be up, too, but psychiatry is not my area of expertise. I'm not sure what my area is. But what we must consider now is that there are a lot of Americans who are of an age when the libido, testosterone and the urge to attract others sexually is as strong as the virus.

One of my granddaughters is seventeen. Her boyfriend, also of the same age, joins my granddaughter as seniors in high school. They were expecting to attend the Senior Prom and walk across the stage at the Saratoga Performing Arts Center in upstate New York in June along with hundreds of their classmates. Not now. New York State schools are closed until May 15, and no large gatherings are expected to occur the rest of this school year. Wearing masks is de rigueur and, in some places, mandatory. My granddaughter has been seeing her boyfriend on a regular basis for two years, and while I am sure that no pre-marital sex has taken place (Oh, shut up!), hooking up is difficult. The boyfriend pulls up into my granddaughter's driveway and the two converse together while the girlfriend sits on her front steps. Verbal correspondence is taking place while being socially distant. Americans are ingenious.

What must it be like for college-age youth and thirty-somethings? Does the word, 'danger' come to mind? Of course! We already know that e-mail, phones and other electronic devices play their role in keeping people in touch with one another. Tension is relieved, but pent-up emotions are running high. My guess is that sexually-active Americans and others across the world will succumb to "*Vouloir, c'est pouvoir.*" That's how the French would say, 'Where there's a will, there's a way.' I think.

It's Sunday. Any changes? Yep. No one is in church. Social distancing is still in place, and Americans are continuing to adapt. Yesterday, the Air Force Academy in Colorado held its graduation ceremony outdoors. Hundreds of young men and women in uniform, seated the required six feet apart listened to the graduation address given by Vice President, Mike Pence. Pence announced that the next rocket carrying astronauts into space would be American made and be fired from American soil. Future astronauts sitting in the audience applauded the word that the United States was back in the space program. In Washington, some news took place.

On the hospital scene, a new demand has come forth. A need for dialysis machines has been uncovered since the 19 virus attacks the kidneys as well as the lungs and other organs in the body. Planners in the WH Virus Team are working on a schedule to get America back to work, and a 3-phase plan was outlined. The plan would work with regional areas of several states working in conjunction with each other and gradually opening up businesses, schools, restaurants and places where people gather. All this depends on how the apex of the virus looks in each geographical area.

The media is still constantly questioning whether

America is going to hold China accountable for its reluctance to share information on the outbreak of the virus. However, getting anything definite about the source and escape of the disease is like capturing the air in a bottle; you know it's there, but you just cannot be sure. Americans are more frustrated than ever. Protests are strong in some states, Americans want their freedoms back.

It is easy to understand this frustration. Americans are used to being part of huge crowds of people who attend football, baseball, basketball and scores of other sporting events. They are fans of large-audience concerts where they cheer, sing, wave their cell-phone lights and sway to the music of the DMB and other musical groups. Americans are used to movie theaters, political rallies and vacationing at seaside resorts. They are used to being part of large crowds at airline terminals awaiting flights with others...unmasked. Americans have been cooped up, and they have followed directions as to how they are to conduct themselves at home and elsewhere. And, now, after weeks of this imposed social distancing, they are beginning to shout, chant and voice their protestations to elected officials who, like one California politician, our Speaker of the House, opens her $25,000 freezer and scoops out ice cream instead of being in Washington. Hey, that's just something which could not be true. But, let me offer a solution to all this virus scare. Here it is: catch the god-damned virus!

Why not? Have you, mighty reader, ever contracted the flu, a virus, a sore throat or runny nose? Oh, yes, you have. How did you cope with it? When you were young, your parents or guardians gave you cough syrup and flu medicine. You stayed home from school. You slept it off.

You rubbed Vicks Vapor Rub on your chest, and you got rid of the infection. And, yes, you sometimes made a visit to a doctor. As you got older, you might have added a little Jack Daniels to your regimen, but you knew that, no matter what you did, no matter how you treated the malady, getting rid of a cold or virus usually took from seven to fourteen days. Why do you think the specialists working on the White House Virus Program prescribe a fourteen-day waiting period or lockdown for infected patients? Simple. Return to the future. If we are going to lick this thing, let's do it like we used to do it. As for me, an 81-year old, I might not make it. Hell, my Marine Corps Gunny sergeant used to tell me, "Remaley, do you think you are going to live forever?" Let me add one little story about a recent person who tested positive.

In 1967, I had the pleasure of being the head football coach of the Junior Varsity Bradford, PA football team. Given thirty wonderful sophomores all of whom were about sixteen years old, we practiced under the hot August sun and, because of the character of those boys, our team was the co-champion of junior varsity teams in that area. On that team, two twin brothers, Dave and Pete Ross, my quarterback and running back respectively, paved the way for a successful season. Recently, Dave reported to me that both Pete and his wife had just recovered from a bout with the COVID-19 virus. Pete, now a dentist, has high blood pressure, is diabetic and has asthma, all pre-conditions which make catching the virus more lethal. Here's the good news. Both Pete and his wife recovered…at home. The surprising thing is this: Dave and his brother are now in their late 60's. How they could have grown to be older than the old guy who coached them is amazing.

Here we are on a Monday. Were there any breaking news flashes over the weekend? Doesn't happen. The regular Monday-through-Friday talking heads frown on handing over top stories to the 'weekend guy'. Most of the weekend news is made up of reruns and summaries of WH Briefings and political ramblings. For example, the need for PPE's, personal protection equipment, is constant. But, of today's T.V. first responders said that for each patient, masks and gowns had to be changed. Why? If two patients are suffering from the same malady, why would health personnel change equipment that had to be discarded? Doesn't make sense. Neither does this 19 thing.

Hospital beds? The Javits Convention Center in New York and the hospital ship in New York Harbor have hundreds of beds, and most of them are empty. Yet, there is still a clamoring for more. Some of the requested respirators and ventilators are still unused and resting idle. Are Americans starting to rely on home remedies and use their own beds at home? These changes and others are causing some hospitals to worry about paying their bills. No patients are showing up at the ER, and few patients are requesting routine elective surgery. No money coming in is a concern for all first responders, and hospital workers are now experiencing the same difficulties as those who lost their jobs in restaurants, shops and entertainment venues. Rents and mortgages must be paid.

The WH Virus Relief Team has proposed a 3-phase plan which, when implemented, would open places of business on a gradual basis. Americans know that thousands of planes rest idle on tarmacs in the Southwest, an area conducive to less wear and tear on parts and motors. We are now hearing stories about planes landing in JFK with one passenger on board. It is said that one plane landing in Chicago had only eight people as its cargo. A maintenance worker at Sky Harbor Terminal in Phoenix reported that planes are flying, but they are only carrying bundles and packages. However, when you look up into the sky, there are no vapor trails. In my own experience, we, my wife and I, have been bumped off our scheduled flight four times. I am now more eager than ever to record what transfers, check-ins, boarding and in-flight service might be like...or not.

APRIL 21, 2020

What pandemic? Oh, it's still here. Like an open sore which won't heal. Over 42,000 Americans have succumbed to 19, and we are only in the fourth month of the year. However, there are signs that individual Americans are resilient. One high school senior from Iowa is using her time to strengthen her ties with family and classmates by challenging them to rise up and persevere during the crisis. Even a verbal-electronic message of hope can help. Wedding ceremonies are taking place via video conferencing. No one seems to be giving up in this battle against the disease. However, as you might expect, there are some glitches.

In Canada, a small community in Nova Scotia suffered what might have been a breakdown in the stay-at-home order. A man went on a shooting spree and killed 19 (coincidence?) people. Not a good omen. As usual, the man's neighbors swore that the shooter was well liked and a respected member of his community. All too often, comments like that are expected, and they ward off unwanted criticism.

Elsewhere in the world, the price of oil has dropped to $11.00 a barrel, and such a cost reflects a production war between oil-producing nations and a dropping demand for petroleum. The airlines are not putting planes in the air, and Americans are not taking long trips to exotic places by automobile. One person joked, "My car has gone one month without filling up." Ocean cruises are no longer popular, and the mass illnesses on board ships has darkened the desire to sail the waves with hundreds of others.

Cabin fever is again playing a role in how Americans react to sheltering-in-place. Demonstrations and protests against social distancing and not working are taking place. Such an outcry has pushed Washington to call for and put into place a 3-phase plan for reopening America. Under this plan, a gradual reopening would take place with individual states leading the way if a flattening of the testing positive curve takes place. May 1 has been set as a possible beginning for a reopening. However, a resurgence of the virus could put a stop to any move. And, if a resurgence were to take place, a political spear would be thrown at the White House from the opposition.

The China syndrome? Oh, yeah. Politicians are still pointing fingers at the experiments which allegedly took place in a Wuhan laboratory. An investigation into the matter has been called for. However, reality tells me that we would not get as much out of an investigation into China's culpability, and it would end up on the floors of Congress like the investigation into 9/11. Remember anything which came out of that? Me either.

Take a break! Breathe in…slowly. Now, breathe out. That's it! Last evening on our AZ patio, Marilyn, my wonderful wife and companion for sixty-one great years, enjoyed a glass (Ok, two) of white and red wine. As we so, we noticed how nature was coping with 19. Clear blue skies, and no vapor trails told us that the air was healthy, and not one cloud broke the solid blue above us. While we do not have the communitive skills of Dr. Doolittle, we watched as multi-colored humming birds, mourning doves, woodpeckers and bunnies were going about the business of doing what they do. The foraged for food, and since, it is spring, they were in the various stages of procreating and caring for their young. Our feathered and furry friends were oblivious of the calamity taking place in the world of humans. Those little creatures imitate us humans, but they don't have time to sense human fears. The sight of that lack of concern for things human was refreshing.

Now, the bad stuff. President Trump has called for immigration to be temporarily suspended. Accepting newcomers onto our soil is not the appropriate thing to do at the moment. Democrats immediately called the decision to keep potentially-positive virus people out of the country a racist move. Hum? There is a downward trend to numbers of Americans testing positive from the virus. In other news, a second relief package designed to help small businesses is being discussed in Congress. That body of working or non-working politicians is painfully slow. An oil glut has caused the price of a barrel of oil to drop dangerously low. But, in spite of the low cost of fuel, airlines are experiencing financial difficulty. No one wants to be cramped in an airliner with those who might test positive, and people know that the air in the cabin is circulated, but not filtered carefully.

Now, about this testing thing. Weeks ago, it was a lack of respirators and ventilators. Then, we, America, did not have enough PPE's. Now, it's a shortage of testing materials. There seems to be a constant whine concerning what is needed, and some of the clamoring is directed at the COVID-19 Task Force. The blame game is heated. Look, there is a fifteen-minute test, a five-minute test, a two or three-day test. There is a swab test, a shine-a-light on your forehead and take-your-temperature test. There is a false-negative test, an antibodies test and a self-diagnosis test. People in the medical field as well as non-medically trained politicians who are calling for all 350 million Americans to be tested…twice. After it (the testing) is done, if a person is found to be negative for the virus, he or she goes down the street and encounters a friend who sneezes. Back to testing. Back to washing your hands, not touching your face and wearing a mask. Around and around we go and where we end up, nobody knows.

Why not make and follow a plan? Associate with only those you know or live or work. If you need to go outside that circle of intimates, wear a god-damned mask…until it's over. Here's an example of that plan which works. Last week, one of my bicycle tires developed a flat. No problem. Take the tire to the bike shop for repair. Hey, the shop was open! But social distancing was in practice. Customers were lined up separated by the six-foot distance, and they were called into the shop one by one. Sales took place, the needed repairs were described. Three days later, I returned to the shop to pick up my now usable tire. Same procedure. One by one, customers were served, and more importantly, employees of the bike shop were earning a living in an efficient, safe way. In other words, where there's a will, there's a way. One thing was noticeable in the shop; not one of the employees was wearing a mask. Oh, well.

Hey, let me rant a little. It's my birthday, and I've lived long enough to say what I feel. Let me use a worn-out phrase, "I have my rights!" OK, now that's over, let's see. What is the source of all this rancor and acrimonious hatred of the American President? Oh, come on. He won. Get over it. Partisan politics is part of it, of course. Devotion to party lines and dogma is another. But, the hostility toward Donald J. Trump borders on insanity.

Yes, I voted for Trump, and I will again. But I also voted for John F. Kennedy and his running mate, Lyndon Johnson. However, we are now at war with an invisible, lethal enemy, COVID-19, and instead of being united against this menace, America is witnessing a childlike behavior by members of Congress and politicians in positions of leadership. These same naysayers are backed by a liberal media, and that is a deadly partnership.

From the first moments of his election as President, there has been a never-ending effort to not only tarnish Trump's reputation but his family's as well. Even his youngest son is not safe from ridicule. Trump has been accused of high crimes and misdemeanors and impeached by members of Congress who, they themselves, have been called out but not prosecuted for insider trading. Adam Schiff, the same House of Representative member who led the impeachment process, has recently proposed that another investigation be made alleging that the President mishandled the 19 debacle. So much for such a childlike complaint. Is there no end to this friction and bitterness in our country? And, the majority of the American media are part of this mob mentality.

An example of political bias and media disruption took place recently when the President called for a temporary halt to immigration. In an effort to keep our borders from being crossed by those who might have the virus, the President called for a slowing of the entry into the United States from abroad. Cries of "Racist", "Xenophobia" rose up immediately from all sides of the opposition. Then, the Governor of the State of New York, Andrew Cuomo, indicated that poor planning was the cause of so much devastation from 19. This is coming from the leader of the state where so much contagion and death occurred. Cuomo also criticized the lack of PPE's, something the previous administration should have covered. Ah, but media blindness covers those tracks. 'Not enough beds!' 'Not enough ventilators!' 'First responders overworked!' And, on it goes.

At the moment, the President is working on getting Americans back to work, a necessary part of the defense to keep our economy safe. Hum? Too early to tell. But, we can all guess what complaints will arise, and among those wishes will not be, "Happy Birthday".

APRIL 24, 2020

What's up today? Well, if you are an elected leader of any country, you are automatically the bullseye of the opposition and the media. Huh? Sure. Boris Johnson, the Prime Minister of the U.K., has just been accused of mishandling the entire coronavirus circus. Surprise, surprise! In Israel, that country's Prime Minister is also under scrutiny. Results of the virus? Perhaps. Johnson was an actual victim of the disease, but he recovered. Although he might have been scarred in his battle with the beast, people are unmoved; he should have ducked!

In other news, Al Gore, one of our former VP's, has endorsed Joe Biden for president in the 2020 race. Biden has yet to choose a running mate. That will give the talking heads something to chew on for a short while. Oh, Harvard University has just received a large amount of money which came from the Virus Relief Package. The school is being asked to return the money since its endowments rival the United States Treasury. Our chances of seeing that money returned to the people are as good as a call for China to pay reparations for its role in covering up the effects of COVID-19. Can you believe it? Some U.S. legislators actually called for China to pay the cost of damage and death to the United States and other countries in its mishandling (there's that word again) of the crisis. I'm sure China will admit guilt in the spread of the virus and it will erase the American national debt in one full payment. And, the Moon and that green cheese thing will happen, too.

On the home front, funerals are taking place without mourners and loved ones who are practicing social distancing. Tyson Foods, the nation's largest pork producer and distributor has suspended plant operations because of low-worker turnout, and that has brought criticism from local Iowans who blame the company for large outbreaks of the virus. President Trump has suggested opening public lands and national parks for Americans seeking to reduce their cabin fever. I wonder what CNN and the media mob will say about that.

T.V. watching? A lot of that is taking place. Not at our home. This morning, two days before our scheduled departure for NY, our cable company jumped the gun and turned off the signal two days before our flight. Oh, well, no big thing. Too many commercials lately, and we still have Wi-Fi. So, in the next two days, there will be a hiatus in the reporting of things encountered by Americans. I am interested in outlining what airline travel is like during the closedown. What will it be like—getting to the airport, checking baggage, going through the TSA checkpoints, boarding the plane, seating arrangements, transfers and final destination landing? I wonder if the Shadow knows. I used to hear that he knew everything.

One more thing before tomorrow's trip. I cannot let this pass since it shows a resiliency in how some people are coping with 19. My daughter, Janine, left high school and went on to get her bachelor's and master's degree in elementary education. She soon married and raised two children, and while doing so, began a business of caring for pre-school children whose parents taught in the local schools. Doing so allowed Janine to enjoy the same schedule as teachers; snow days, holidays, stoppages of any kind allowed Janine and her children time together, that is, until COVID-19 came to town in early April.

From the moment children were no longer coming to Janine's home and while teachers were at home sheltering-in-place, my daughter saw an opportunity to keep learning as part of the shut-in. Videos were made with the help of Janine's son. One such film had a puppet-like Aladdin, the genie handing a bored Janine a magic mirror. With the aid of that mirror, Janine spoke to and greeted each one of her day-care children. Games were played, familiar backyard places were visited and questions asked. Education had not shut down thanks to electronic hookups and CD making. One little glitch did take place. Contracts had been signed at the beginning of the school year stipulating that shutdowns, snow days and holidays were paid periods of time. Since teachers were receiving their full pay during the stay-at-home period of time, day-care center entrepreneurs would receive the same. You know, even during the trying time of this ravaging disease, only one teacher did not hold to the agreement. One out of five or six is still not bad. Good for you, Janine. By the way, your explaining to the one parent that she had to do what was right for her family says much for your devotion.

I wonder what the flight will be like tomorrow.

Here we go, off into the wild, blue yonder, a distant place… maybe. It is 3:10 A.M., Mountain Time, and my wife and I are waiting for our 4:15 pickup to take us to Sky Harbor Airport in Phoenix. Sure, there are questions. Will our shuttle driver be on time? Will we catch our 6:30 flight to Chicago, our connection change of planes? What will we encounter at TSA?

Let's begin. Right on time. Our shuttle arrived, we loaded up our luggage into an eight-seater van. We were the only passengers to the airport, and we arrived in plenty of time for our flight. We arrived at what seemed to be an abandoned building. In a check-in area usually crammed with children, animals, and other adults, we numbered along with other morning flyers about twenty people. We checked our bags as did other masked individuals with the baggage handlers who were also part of a masked mob. It was hard to understand what we were told to do; tongues do not always work well tangled up in cloth-like coverings. I wonder if stagecoach drivers had trouble with desperadoes like Jesse James who, at gunpoint said, "Give me all your Reece Peanut Butter cups." Well, criminal activity back then might have been misinterpreted.

Once given direction to our gate, we headed for the TSA entry area. Once again, masked personnel urged us to stand on socially distant circles on the floor and wait to be given the nod to continue forward. We, too, made up the little group edging forward, and things moved quickly. TSA checked our faces with appropriate picture ID's, but they must have had x-ray vision to see through our masks. We didn't ask them how they were able to see so well.

At our boarding gate, D2, about twenty other passengers, most masked, some not, waited for the 6:30 A.M. departure for Chicago. Our flight had not been cancelled. So, how about a Starbucks coffee and a roll? Are you kidding? Nothing open, no baristas, *nada!* No food, no coffee, no luck. Must be the lockdown. Such a scene brings to mind the fact that a lot of people, those who don't make a lot of money, are out of work. One of the plane's captains checked himself through the gate. He wore no mask. I'd know him anywhere.

At the appropriate moment, flight attendants announced that lines would form for boarding, and we took our places alongside numbered poles. About sixty people, one dog, and one cat in a carryon bag waited patiently. In a machine designed to carry over two hundred passengers, today's flight would have only sixty humans and two animals. The animals wore no masks. Makes you wonder how long Southwest and other airlines will remain in business.

On the three hour and fifty-minute flight to Chicago, flight attendants, all face-covered, served no peanuts, pretzels nor any liquid refreshments. Passengers were seated as normal, but only two to a three-seat row. The first three rows on both sides of the plane were taped off to passengers.

Oh, the cat. You know, the one about the size of a javelina. Well, it protested its being sheltered-in-place, and it did so vehemently throughout the three and a half-hour flight. I love cats. Its meow was like some loud bull-horn announcing a fire alarm. Can cats carry the 19 thing? Dr. Fauci things so. I'm going to invent a freeze-dry spray for such situations. You simply spray your animal or kids, they go to sleep, then you splash them with water, and they return to the living. I'll make a million! The flight turned out to be turbulent, and with every bump, the cat turned up the volume. It is always bumpy flying into the Windy City.

OK, what do you think about when you are 32,000 feet over Kansas, and you are surrounded by fifty or sixty face-covered strangers? I'll tell you what. You suddenly realize that you are not only sheltered-in-place like the cat, you are being held hostage by some politician or scientist who thought it best that you be restrained. You cannot go for a walk, ride a bike, go shopping, take in a movie (I didn't have a note pad or computer with me), and you certainly are not going to enjoy a meal or a nice Bordeaux. You are closed off completely from life such as it was. Then, you start thinking about that little evil bug which started all this—19.

Remember seeing all those hooded and face-covered scientists working with test tubes, looking into microscopes and putting petri dishes into whirly-gig machines? Thinking back, those often-repeated T.V. clips were probably years old, survivors of other viruses. Will a vaccine ever be developed to ward off this thing in months to come? From all that we hear, the chances of such a thing being invented are not good. COVID-19 Task Force doctors don't offer much hope. 'Fall' is beginning to have an ominous meaning.

We have been in the air for only two and a half hours. Still an hour and a half to go. The cat is going strong. I think I'll buzz one of the flight attendants and order a bottle of Cocobon Dark. Oops! They, the face-covered Southwest flight attendants, are seated sheltered-in-place like the rest of us. Maybe later. Maybe not.

Chicago. Windy, wobbling landing. But we arrived. Familiar territory. But I have never seen O'Hare Airport this empty. About sixty travelers patiently wait on our flight to Albany. At an empty restaurant bar, I find a customer counter just right to pen a few observations. We, the masked ones, have about an hour and a half before takeoff. What else is worth documenting?

First of all, here in Chicago and as far as I can see, Americans are adhering to the wearing of protective masks. All but Southwest pilots and some airport service personnel are taking this thing seriously. 'Our masks are better than your masks' seems to be the silent message today. Flowered masks, paisley masks, tie-dye masks, stars and stripes masks make up a sea of multi-colored faces. Our masks, mine and my wife's are better than our unrecognizable travel companions'. Ours are patriotic ones. There is something else, too. In the past, in the large crowds of travelers at airports, one would see all types of exotic dress. Burkas, sarongs, Muslim headdress and sombreros announced many foreign travelers. Not now. Most of the travelers appear to be Americans of fifty years or older. Racist!

Another add on. Southwest pilots, as observed earlier, those waiting for their planes, do not wear masks. Probably former military. That might explain why so many navy personnel are now coming down with the virus. They could never catch 19; they are ten feet tall and bullet proof.

Second leg—our flight out of Chicago. Another observation: now that Americans are covering their faces and hands and the entire body covered in tight-fitting clothing, you cannot distinguish any race or national origin. Hallelujah! Racism is over. Wouldn't that be great! We then would be able to say, "Take that you wily old virus!" There's the call for us to board the plane.

Once on board, something else drew my attention. You know those company-owned magazines found in the pouch of the seat in front of you. They're gone. It might have been the source of too many hands on them, but something else comes to mind. Fewer hotels, restaurants and gadget sellers are advertising. No one is scheduling cruises or vacationing in Las Vegas these days.

Now, what will it be like back in upstate New York? Sure, same old routine. Social distancing, sheltering-in-place, hording toilet paper, standing on little circles six feet apart from the next person, no movies theaters open, no Dunkin Donuts. Oh, well, tomorrow or Monday, we can get back to Task Force Briefings, media misunderstandings, Americans out of work and White House efforts to harness the beast. Not a pretty picture. Learn anything on the trip? Too much!

The final segment of this return to New York has to do with our daughter, Janine. She met us at the airport. No hugs. She, too, was masked. We drove north to Saratoga and tried to interpret conversations interrupted by cloth and tongue twisting. We were instructed to take off our clothes and put them in the wash as soon as we got home, take a shower and then sit down to a dinner Janine had prepared for us. I had not considered the shower. Although it was Saturday, my shower day, it was explained that we had spent the day sitting in airplane seats which had many people there before us. New Yorkers take death seriously. That evening at dinner, we learned that New York State is in lockdown. You don't go anywhere without a mask. Ain't it great! But, at dinner/happy hour, I discussed an idea with Janine and *Madame.*

I discussed the once popular social greeting of shaking hands. Meeting close friends or upon making new ones, Americans used to shake hands. Not now. But old habits are hard to break. So, I suggested making thin plastic hands cut from some kind of soft material which, when cut, could be placed, hooked on and held in place at the end of a three-foot thin wooden dowel. Another person with such a stick could touch hands and say, "High five" of "Hey, there." I'm thinking "Socially-distant hands". After all, three plus three makes six. Good to be home.

APRIL 26, 2020

Here we go again. Death from 19 in the United States has now risen to over 54,000, and it is predicted to reach or surpass 100,000 by fall. Dr. Birx, one of the COVID-19 Task Force members, says that social distancing could last through the summer. On the other hand, states such as Tennessee, Alabama and Georgia are already considering opening on a gradual scale with small businesses operating such as beauty salons, barber shops and other small concerns.

From Washington, VP Pence reports that there are very positive signs of a leveling off and a flattening of the curve of positive tested individuals. President Trump, still besieged by the liberal press, has hinted that future press conferences will be fewer since most questions are negative in nature concerning the Task Force's efforts. The White House briefings are, he says, just a platform for criticism rather than reporting progress.

China is still being credited with having held back critical information which, if shared, could have alerted many nations about the seriousness of the disease. So much for futile gests and talk about reparations from that Asian country.

On the medical front, 'contact tracing' is now being

touted as one of the more useful testing measures. In this procedure, trained staff interviewers talk to those who have been diagnosed with a contagious disease to figure out who they might have encountered during their illness. Then, the staffers go tell the people they may have been exposed to and sometimes encourage them to quarantine themselves to prevent spreading the disease further. Makes me think of the cat on the flight from Phoenix; "Oh, no, not the box again!"

This morning, another interesting aspect of this lockdown occurred. Needing some items from my local hardware store, I called my Ace Hardware store and asked about the procedure of possibly getting the materials needed. A store worker told me that he would take my order, find it and total it while I waited. A few minutes later, the employee confirmed the order, took payment via credit card and told me to come to the store and pull into the parking lot. I followed orders. A masked employee came to my car, authenticated my identity (hard to do with a face cover) and returned to the store and picked up my order, returned and placed it in my care. Customers do not go in the store. That transaction lasted but a few minutes. It was faster, more efficient, saved me time, and people were able to continue working while observing mitigation. How do you say, "Shopping in the future will be different"?

One more entry. The American military and its training of raw recruits is now faced (oops, wrong word) with a new problem. Trainees are now forced to wear PPE's and observe social distancing. During bayonet drills, that could be cumbersome. Remembering my Marine boot camp experiences, a D.I.'s face could express a thousand words. Now, those D.I.'s are masked. Takes some of the fun out of it.

APRIL 27, 2020

What will be learned from today's encounter with the enemy? There's always something. During our early-morning coffee and watching the news, my wife and I were told that the Democrat's candidate for President, Joe Biden, is under pressure to choose a running mate…or give up the quest to even run himself. It was hinted that there might be NFL football at the end of the summer. How that might take place with all the mitigation rules was not divulged.

Throughout the world, thousands are still dying from complications of the virus. China? That country must have eradicated 19 completely from Chinese soil or be masking the truth. Nah! Couldn't happen. Nameless political and media officials are calling for China to come clean and admit its roll in a virus cover up. I am sure that China will fess up and pay the trillions of dollars in reparations demanded by a disgruntled world. Maybe not.

In North Korea, Kim Jong Un, the leader of that communist country, is said to be ill. I hope it's not the virus. It is sometimes lethal. Who knows? Kim's sister is the heir apparent but will she be allowed to live? Kim's relatives have a way of gaining weight from too much lead. I'll ask Nancy Pelosi. She hates men…well, Donald Trump anyway. She wears such decorative masks.

Americans are calling for a May opening of certain businesses. Barber shops, beauty salons and other small enterprises will open in certain states late this month and early in May. That move, of course, will be contested loudly by those who still have a salary. Do members of Congress come to mind? Health-conscious Americans are eager to start working out again. Our "Y", now closed and showing empty parking lots used to be packed all hours of the day. Not anymore.

Been to a bank lately? It had been my custom to go inside my bank and do business. My bank and others have locked their doors, but drive-ups are open. Pneumatic tubes now take our money, and I am reminded of seeing those machines in department stores in the 1940's. No smart remarks about age; we're in a crisis here! Grocery stores? *Madame et moi* did our first New York State shopping inside our local market this morning. We had some restocking to do since we just returned from a sunny Southwest yesterday. All shoppers and supermarket personnel wore masks. The now familiar socially-distant circles on the floor helped us to avoid mistakes. Ah, our store also had neatly-painted arrows showing us which aisles to enter and which to not. Those directional aids give you more space since you usually don't encounter a fellow shopper going the wrong way. Well, almost. There is always that ten percent who don't get the word or those who do not know the story of the Yellow-brick road.

Did I say that the second relief package, that designed to keep small business afloat, starts today? I wonder if Harvard will get a big stimulus. I think I'll go press my mask. It's a little wrinkled. Tomorrow? A new and effective vaccine? More calls for testing? Hey, one out of two ain't bad.

'Asymptomatic', presenting no symptoms of disease is now one of the important words used to indicate how one should look at 19. Dr. Birx, now a well-known spokesperson in the fight against the virus, warns Americans that masks are still a good idea in keeping the disease in check. People who have no outward symptoms of the sickness could unknowingly spread the virus to others in public. As if to add weight to the argument and Dr. Birx's advice, Jet Blue Airlines has now issued a directive that all future passengers on its planes will be required to wear face coverings.

In the area of testing, the antibodies tests are coming into question. Those who have been infected with 19 and recovered once thought that they could not again become infected because of the antibodies produced in their system might have resulted in immunity. Not so, reports some scientists. Further investigation is needed on the subject. People are advised to pay attention to the symptoms: chills, aches, fevers, repeated shaking, sneezing, coughing and muscle pain.

There is a movement and demand from some states such as Georgia, Oklahoma, Tennessee and others to reopen their economies on a gradual basis. Small businesses are especially hard hit by the requested shutdowns, and from what we have learned about the efficiency of certain grocery stores, hardware stores and other small enterprises, Americans can go back to earning a living. However, mitigation is de rigueur; masks and social distancing are required. There has been an overwhelming request from small business owners for increased funds needed to enable them to continue to pay their employees. In fact, the federal system of distributing such funds is breaking down because of the high demand for help.

In foreign news, it has been reported that North Korea's leader, Kim Jong Un, is in critical condition after what might have been an accident occurring during a missile shot or a botched operation in a hospital. No accurate account of his condition is coming out of that communist country. How strange! Many other countries are still asking that China pay for their economic losses because of possible Chinese cover ups. Let me see...

American hospitals are in serious financial difficulty because no elective surgeries have been taken place in those institutions, and bills have to be paid. The intensive care of COVID-19 patients has taken precedence over general needs, and the demand for PPE's has taken a lot of money. Let's see what transpires in the next twenty-four hours. Here, in upstate New York, sunshine. How unusual.

By the way, in the light of what we Americans are going through, it just might be a good idea to reach out electronically, by phone, Skype or some other safe method, and tell someone and/or those you love that you miss them and wish them well. Doesn't cost much, and a lot of people could use a kind gesture right now. Already done that? Do it again.

A beautiful sight took place yesterday over New York, New Jersey and Pennsylvania. In a salute to health-care workers and first responders, an 'America Strong' show of support and appreciation was offered in a fly-over by the Air Force Thunderbirds and the Navy's Blue Angels. Thousands of hospital workers, firemen and police flooded the streets down below and enjoyed the display of strength in the air. The smiles and applause recorded on T.V. gave proof that Americans have not lost hope.

In other news, Hillary Clinton endorsed Joe Biden for President. The former Secretary of State also expressed her desire for a national health-care plan, something which will end up in the Democrat's platform later this year. Mr. Biden is now being accused of sexual harassment by a woman with whom he worked while in the Senate. Media moguls are slow to question the presidential candidate on the matter, and political bias is being shown once again. One thinks back to the coverage of Bret Kavanagh and his nomination for a seat on the Supreme Court under similar circumstances. Political bias? No way.

Chinese scientists now predict that the COVID-19 virus might never disappear and that it will return in waves. This same group admits that an experiment developing infectious diseases did take place in its labs in Wusan, but no admission of guilt in its escape was mentioned. No consideration of paying other countries for the damage caused to economies and human beings was offered. I was sure that China would do the right thing…and that the Saratoga Thoroughbred will open this summer where thousands of race goers spend lots of money. Hum.

Every academic year, thousands of Chinese students are sent to the United States by their government to study the latest scientific and economic trends. Some of those trends are secret, and I am sure they do not ever carry such information back to their native country. Do they? Shouldn't it be time for the United States to question such practices? No. Not as long as our universities accept huge payments for tuition, room and board. Chances are good that such practices will not end soon.

More and more Americans are going outside a protesting their 'quarantine fatigue.' Walking, running, exercising, bathing and taking in the fresh air will probably increase. However, these health-conscious Americans do wear masks. That's good. Dr. Fauci and Dr. Birx would be proud. Along with the outdoors activities, many Americans are beginning to support opening up businesses. They want to earn a paycheck again. The federal PPP program's round 2 starts this week, and the Paycheck Protection Program will help thousands of American pay their bills for another two weeks.

By the end of today, 60,000 Americans will have died from 19. Some of those who lost loved ones to the disease are now filing law suits against employers who allegedly did not do enough to protect workers. The expression, "It was not their fault", sums up what might weaken such legal efforts. The virus is an equal-opportunity killer.

On the bright side, today is my son's birthday. That he is among the living, that he served his country as a United States Marine, and that he has been a good father to his children brings pleasure to me and his mother. I will call him later and tell him what I just told you. Find a reason to express your love for someone today. It will make you part of 'America Strong.'

Reader, are you working today? Are you putting in an eight-hour day earning a wage? You might be one of the lucky Americans gainfully employed. If you are like almost 15 percent of the workforce, you might be receiving unemployment insurance payments. But, the majority of our elected officials in Washington are not working. Yes, they are getting paid and enjoying insider-trading benefits. Ever hear anything about the four members of Congress accused of but not prosecuted for such a thing? Nope. Me either. Senators and House members of Congress are getting paid, but they are now at home unwilling to encounter the chance of testing positive for the virus. Did those more-equal Americans suggest a pay cut during this tragedy? I must have missed that. Might be time for term limits.

Yesterday, 330 New Yorkers died from the virus. Governor Cuomo has just mandated that New York State residents will wear masks, and that he will rely on data as to whether or not small business will reopen. I wonder if I should give him a call (Skype, of course), and tell him that hardware stores, supermarkets, auto-repair shops and certain take-out restaurants are open for business across New York State. Ah, he probably already knows that.

Good news. Germany has some positive evidence that their scientists might be close to producing a vaccine to ward off the virus. Although more testing in that country and in the United States will be required, at least there is some hope that a defensive preparation might be forthcoming.

At home, here in Saratoga and in towns and cities throughout the country, America's students, secondary as well as college, are wondering whether their classes will resume this year. My granddaughter, a high-school senior would like to attend the senior prom with her boyfriend, a senior at her school. Both of them look forward to walking across the stage of the Saratoga Performing Arts Center in June and receiving their high-school diploma. My granddaughter is also wondering what her freshman year at Potsdam State and her volleyball games will be interrupted. Here and across the country, such anxiety is pent up but held in check. Hell, they are Americans.

Whatever the case, schools will perhaps never be the same. When I taught, students enrolled in my high school and university classes would change classes at a specific time. Hundreds and sometimes even thousands of students would fill the hallways and jostle for position while going to their next classroom. Cafeterias were crowded knee to knee at lunch tables which held eight to ten students. Even with faces covered, such things would not be appropriate at the moment. And, teaching will never be the same with twenty or more students sitting at desks two feet apart.

Purdue University's President recently stated that school calendars will change state by state, and that the art of teaching will never be the same. However, some American events might see a return. Will we hear in late spring the once familiar chant, "Play ball!"? Major League Baseball is now investigating how the game could be played. College and professional football and every other sport admired and encouraged by sports-loving Americans will face the same situation—to play or not to play. Can we Americans live without sportscasters saying, "Watch this rerun of that play! She could be the next All-American volleyball player from Potsdam State."? Hey, this is my book! I'm not interested in an editor telling me that I cannot tout my granddaughter's undergraduate school. I hope it opens this fall.

Michael Flynn redux! Why would anyone want to bring Flynn back to the future? He had nothing to do with the 19 thing. Maybe so, but intrigue and mystery surrounding the man's trials and tribulations are worth a look. They might throw light on the reluctance of some Democrats to support America's fight against the virus. It must be admitted that partisan politics has played a role in weakening a needed solidarity in our war with the contagion. Let's start with the period of time immediately before the 2016 presidential election.

In August of 2016, months before Donald Trump was elected President, Peter Strzok was having an affair with Lisa Page, an FBI lawyer. Strzok told his lover, Page, "We'll stop Donald Trump from becoming President." Page replied, "Trump's not ever going to be President, right? Right?" Strzok's answer was, "No, no, he won't." Hum! Sounds a little like some kind of prejudice, doesn't it. Now, how were these two lovebirds and their associates, all Trump haters, going to carry this off? Enter James B. Comey and his FBI cohorts.

James Comey, using his position as Director of the FBI, discovered that Michael Flynn, President Trump's National

Security Advisor, had recently traveled to Russia and had spoken to Russian security agents on the matter of terrorism. Flynn, the retired Army three-star general, was about to step into a quicksand bed, and unfortunately, he trusted the FBI not yet aware of the 'deep state' existence of former Obama appointees.

Strzok and others in his gang were sent to the White House after a meeting with Flynn had been set up. At that meeting, Flynn was promised by the FBI agents that only terrorism would be discussed and that White House lawyers would not be necessary. Flynn gave his approval, and the meeting took place between the fly and the spider. It has often been said by those who know the law that anyone can be maneuvered into telling a lie, especially when questioned by FBI lawyers. At the meeting, Flynn divulged that he had spoken to Russian officials but that he remembers little about the specifics. One thing took place after another, and Flynn was accused of lying to FBI agents about the contents of the meeting with the Russians. Wiretaps might have convinced the lawyers that they knew more than they let on. Flynn was convinced that he should plead guilty to lying, and that, if he did not, his son, a man who had worked with his father, would be brought into the investigation and charged as an accomplice. To protect his son, Flynn pleaded guilty to lying.

The next day, after hearing that his National Security Director had pleaded guilty to lying, President Trump fired Flynn in an effort to cleanse his administration of any wrongdoing. Flynn, a thirty-year veteran of the Army who had served his country, was forced to hire attorneys to protect him from prosecution. In that defense, the general lost his home and was mired in six million dollars of legal debt.

Recently, President Trump's Attorney General and his staff uncovered written notes by Strzok and Page which confirmed that Flynn was set up as a scapegoat. In other evidence against the FBI and its action in the plot, it was revealed that Michael Horowitz, another Clinton supporter and presidential appointee, had conducted an investigation into Flynn's case and stated, "We did not find documentary of testimonial evidence that improper considerations (by the FBI) including political bias, covertly affected the specific investigative actions we reviewed." Right!

As of the present time, May 1, 2020, Michael Flynn still does not know whether he is a free man. James Comey in 2017 bragged to a full-of-laughter audience of media and Clinton backers that he sent Peter Strzok to the White House knowing that he could capitalize on a chaotic place. Adam Schiff, a House of Representative member, further added to the chaos in the White House with his effort to impeach Donald Trump. Now, do you think that there was an opposition to the Trump presidency? Nah! The evil in all this matter rests in the fact that these things took place while a deadly virus crept its way into our heartland. Yet, the naysayers still claim that Trump did not do enough in the early weeks of the outbreak. You know, he has been busy with collusion with the Russians and fighting off impeachment accusations. Just sayin'.

In other news of the day, doctors are warning that vaping and the use of tobacco products does harm the lungs and makes them susceptible to contagion of 19. Joe Biden, like others before him, has been accused of sexual misconduct by a staff member he knew in the late 90's. In an action against the virus, the President has called for a 'warp speed' effort to come up with a vaccine against the virus. The Little League World Series in Williamsport, PA has been cancelled for the first time in history because of complications of testing positive for the virus. On the other hand, NASCAR will run a race in two weeks but without spectators. And, lastly, 30 million Americans are jobless and are not applying for unemployment benefits. Stay safe, wear masks, wash your hands, practice social distancing and shelter-in-place…at least for the time being.

Let's review some of the breaking news. Governor Cuomo just announced that the New York State public schools are closed for the remainder of the academic year. He also advised summer school officials to make efforts to determine how those classes might work and to plan and safely run classes in September. Joe Biden has been accused of sexual harassment by a woman who allegedly had an encounter with Biden in 1993, twenty-seven years ago. Nancy Pelosi immediately came to Biden's defense saying, "Joe Biden is Joe Biden." And, a rose is a rose is a rose. Listeners seemed to take Pelosi's response to mean that the former VP under President Obama is without guilt in this sexual harassment accusation. Female Democrats have said in the past that all women should be believed. Hum?

During the Supreme Court Hearings held during Bret Kavanaugh's nomination for a seat on the court, the cry that all women should be believed was voiced loud and clear by female Senators and Representatives. Will those same women change their tune? Not likely. Do we have a case of the double standard here? Of course; politics are politics. Will anything change or make a difference here? Nope.

Earlier this morning, Biden took part in an interview

on MSNBC's "Morning Joe" program. In that interview, conducted by a female reporter, Biden declared, "It never happened." President Trump, when asked for his opinion on the matter, deftly responded, "I don't know anything about it. It happened to me, too." Let's see what CNN says about the accusation later today.

On the vaccine against the 19 virus, a former Marine friend of mine gave me a call this morning from Florida. He told me that his son, George Morris, a cancer-clinic nurse in Portland, Oregon, had good news concerning the drug Remdesivir. Morris is working with others in his hospital on a serum, not a true vaccine, which when administered, does have a significant positive affect on the disease by reducing the severity of the affliction. Dr. Fauci on the COVID-19 White House Team echoes the findings. How a former Marine's son could have acquired such skills is beyond me. Must be the mother.

We have already discussed air travel, and my recent experience flying cross-country has been documented. In the future, airlines will probably require that all passengers wear masks. Airline attendants will likely not by serving pretzels, peanuts and liquid refreshment up and down the aisles during the flights. That might be a good idea; keeping those passage ways clear would be helpful to everyone needing restroom facilities. Now, other businesses are demonstrating that life and wage earning can go on.

This morning, my wife wanted to know if any stores were open which sold wine. In New York State, supermarkets do not sell any alcohol other than beer. Wanting to keep peace in my sheltered-in-place home, a call was made to our local liquor store, and the clerk was asked to outline procedures for ordering, paying for and picking up whatever the customer wanted. I was told that no one could enter the wine store, but customers could order over the phone, pay by credit card, and when the customer arrived in the store's parking lot, a call could be made alerting the store's personnel that a customer was waiting outside. All this was done. I had ordered two cases of wine—one white, one red. Two cases? Yes, I don't really like the stuff. My wife and I use it as paper weights. Lasts only for a short time. Evaporation in terrible in upstate New York. However, this experience with shopping by phone was super. Going into the store and being tempted by pretty-looking bottles was avoided. Time was saved, efficient shopping was done, and Americans were earning a salary. Works all the way around.

News reports around the Nation and abroad tend to be more- sparse than the Monday through Friday offering. Radio and television owners give their regular hosts the weekend off, and the replacements, the 'weekend guy' is not given scoops to outline to the listening and watching public. Even in the Nation's Capital, things change during the Saturday/Sunday period. Donald Trump will be in the rustic retreat at Camp David. The President's entourage will complete a working weekend there.

Rumors, even in times of strife and crisis, abound. Some Americans are implying that deaths attributed to COVID-19 are perhaps artificially inflated. One individual, a woman in Florida, claims that her husband recently died at home from cardiac arrest. The county coroner signed the death certificate of the husband and declared the cause of death to be the coronavirus. Similar stories can be found throughout the United States, and some people hint that the inflated figures relating to the virus might have to do with monetary allocations to states or cities with high death rates from the contagion. New York State and New York City? Nah! Such reports could produce panic or disgust in the country. Wait! It already has.

Throughout the nation, Americans are protesting stay-at-home orders, and they want to go outside and enjoy the public parks and beaches. Florida and California seaside resorts are now witnessing beach goers in large numbers defying the shutdown of such places. In Detroit, Michigan's Governor has been chastised for her reluctance to open her state to business as usual. All across America, business owners are starting to take matters into their own super-washed hands and open their shop doors on a partial and safe basis.

Some decisions made by other U.S. state governors are now in question. California's Governor recently released from prison over 3,000 violent criminals into the general population. Californians were told that these former prisoners were in jeopardy of contracting the virus. Unfortunately, some of these newly-released law breakers have once again committed felonies, and some of them have tested positive for the virus, thus making them carriers of the disease. What causes such elected officials to disregard the law-abiding Americans over convicted criminals? Politics? Couldn't be.

The anti-viral drug, Remdesivir, is getting good press. The administering of this drug is said to have sped up recovery from the disease and make symptoms less harmful to the body. Elsewhere, meat processing plants are closing because of high rates of testing positive by those in the workplace. Meat shortages have been predicted, and political activists are calling for the President to impose the Nation's Defense Production Act. It must be Trump's fault that our meat-processing plant workers are prone to coming down ill. "Not enough PPE's!" Let me see. Where have I heard that before?

In other business areas, Elon Musk, the builder of the Tesla automobile, has come forward with his new, less expensive model. However, he cannot get permission to reopen his plant in spite of orders flying off the roof. Musk, like other American entrepreneurs, wants America to get back to work.

Now, one last but important thing in today's message. Remember the 1st Paycheck Protection Program stimulus? Under that proposal, and injection of cash directly into the hands of Americans whose yearly income was less than $125,000.00, would receive $1,200.00 to help pay weekly and monthly bills. *Madame et moi* were recipients of that stipend. Our income was under the max…way under. But, more importantly, our daughter and her husband received the same amount. That is important because my daughter is a health-care provider for children of parents who are teachers. Schools closed, my daughter was no longer employed, and that sum of money will help in so many ways. Most of that money will go immediately back into the economy. Congress and, yes, the President and his task force, need to be congratulated on such foresight. Will they be? Maybe.

Now, let's see. The Senate is working, but the House, instructed by its Leader, Nancy Pelosi, is staying away from Washington and sheltering-in-place. Joe Biden's accuser of sexual harassment, Tara Reade, is still proclaiming abuse from an incident which occurred in 1993. The 'Me, too' movement Democrats, women who believe women, have moved away from any opinion on the matter, and the silence they are expressing is loud and clear—partisan. In my opinion, Reade should let sleeping dogs lie; not to have expressed her concern years ago in an appropriate way does smack of seeking attention.

On Saturday, the Kentucky Derby did not take place… well, not in the sense of seeing thoroughbreds crashing around a track. However, electronics and a computer-generated version of the race did take place. No great audience of race goers were on hand, but in that electronically-generated race, Secretariat did come out the winner. In Spain, another sporting event fell to the virus. The famous 'Running of the bulls at Pamplona' was cancelled. The thousands of onlookers at that special happening were not present, and tourism throughout Europe is absent. Economic panic has not yet set in, but without the millions of pleasure seekers,

Europe will suffer. Even the 'Tour de France' has been postponed. *Mon dieu!*

As far as remedies for the COVID-19 virus, Remdesivir is being discussed. Dr. Birx has stated that the drug is not a silver bullet, but, in some cases, it has lessened the severity of the illness. She, one of the members of the President's Virus Task Force, says that Americans need to continue to mitigate and use social distancing. She also says that wearing masks does not automatically ensure that no contagion will take place.

Across the Nation, ten states have shut down all religious gatherings. Beaches in some states have been declared closed, and that has led to protests by pent-up Americans. The danger of too many people deciding to open their doors and step outside for recreation and enjoyment might lead to more than 140,000 deaths.

In Washington yesterday, another virtual happening took place at the Lincoln Memorial. President Trump met with representatives from Fox News and answered questions from Americans across the United States on matters relating to the virus and life as it is. That Virtual Town Meeting might have helped ease America's mind, but the disease is still with us. Discussed at the meeting was how we will possibly open our economy and continue the fight against 19. In another item, some cities throughout America are asking for aid and bailouts concerning their debts run up over the past decades. Many believe that those cities do not deserve such consideration because outrageous pension plans have devastated their budgets.

Cinco de mayo! Before the 19 thing hit the United States, Americans would end the day by stopping in bars and restaurants and celebrate something having to do with Mexico. They didn't care that the date is the commemoration of Mexico's defeat of Napoleon III's army at the battle of Pueblo in 1867. The day was a time to let loose and take advantage to drink beer. I'll bet that not much of Corona beer will be consumed today. Most bars and restaurants are now closed, but there is a move in some states to reopen.

Remember my story of phone shopping at my local hardware? Here's a redux on that anecdote. After ordering what I needed by phone, I made the mistake of not checking for understanding before hanging up. Always ask the person on the other end of the line to confirm verbally what you have ordered. If not, you are more than likely to be missing some of the things you needed when the order is picked up. That happened to me, and it is always a good idea to have a cell phone with you when you arrive in the store's parking lot. Once you arrive, call the store and let them know that you are outside. Otherwise, you might waste a lot of time thinking someone will not be aware of your presence. No one goes into the store.

In San Francisco yesterday, there was a problem with police personnel wearing masks. Officers had been using white and black masks depicting the American stars and stripes which they called, "Blue line" masks. The Chief of Police of the above city declared that the masks might be seen as an association to the administration in Washington. Can't have politics enter into the fight against the virus!

Airlines are struggling as to how to stay in business. Some companies are requiring all passengers to wear masks from check in to deplaning. TSA personnel must really be having a tough time—"Sir, are you the person in this picture?" Other airline companies are offering the middle seat empty, but you pay extra for that privilege. When asked whether it was now safe to fly, Dr. Mark Siegel from New York University stated, "Yes, as long as your destination is not an epicenter of the disease. That limits your choices somewhat.

It was also reported that as many as 134,000 American deaths from the disease could occur by August. Those in nursing homes and those with pre-condition diseases such as obesity, diabetes, heart and lung problems are the most susceptible to dying. In response to all this bad news, films shown to the television audience display restaurant workers wiping down menus…restaurants that are open, that is. Grocery stores are now limiting the amount of meat one can buy. Environmentalists and cardiologists will be happy.

Happy *Cinco de Mayo!* And, stay away from the Corona. You never know.

MAY 6, 2020

Over a century ago, a famous writer penned a book entitled, "A Tale of Two Cities". That story rings true today. Bristal, Georgia and Bristal, Tennessee are side-by-side communities divided by an imaginary line and political boundaries. They are both trying to plan out how to deal with the back to work issue. Americans on the Georgia side of the city are ready and willing to get back to work, open businesses and earn a living. The Governor of Tennessee is opposed to getting back to work early. The results of that split decision will be known in weeks to come. Let's wish them both luck.

There is a supposed meat shortage in the United States. Meat processing plants in Iowa and other parts of the nation are now closed because too many workers have tested positive for the 19 virus. Some fast-food restaurants are taking burgers off their menus due to a shortage of the food product. And, of course, some people are suggesting that meat packers are playing games with the economy. Something tells me that some Americans will soon be hoarding meat just like those who piled up toilet paper in their shopping carts in the month of March. Understanding the phenomenon of hoarding escapes me.

The President's Coronavirus Task Force is once again

in the news. One of its members, Dr. Anthony Fauci, has been asked by the House of Representatives Committee on the virus to meet with them and discuss how the war on the disease is being conducted. President Trump, already stung by previous House investigative committees, has suggested that instead of meeting with the House, that the Senate will have that privilege. I'm sure no bias on the part of anyone here played a part in that decision. Aren't you? Another inquiry is certainly not needed. People should be allowed to do their job. Dr. Fauci will meet this week in the Senate where a little more bipartisan meeting might take place.

Why Dr. Fauci? Hum! Recently, Chris Cuomo, a CNN News reporter, contracted the virus. Cuomo, brother to Andrew Cuomo, the Governor of New York, has been the darling of evening newscasts. Doing his show from his home, viewers were able to see firsthand the effects of the disease. More importantly, one of Chris Cuomo's best friends has telephoned the sick man at his home and inquired about his health. The caller? Dr. Anthony Fauci. Now, just why would the House of Representatives be interested in Fauci's opinions on how the President was conducting the war on the virus? Gee, I don't know. I wonder what the good doctor will say to the Senate.

There are now some complications relating to the disease. For some reason, 19 has influenced the spread of Kawasaki's disease, a rare infection that affects the blood vessels in children ages 5 and younger. It just seems to gather speed like a flood sweeping through some valley community.

Mike Huckabee, former Governor of Arkansas, was recently asked whether some Americans were feeling vulnerable about going back to work. He said that those who feel vulnerable should stay at home. Those who don't must make a choice. If you watch the different television channels on whether things are going well with decision making on the virus, an interesting observation can be made. If you are a fan of MSNBC or CNN, you will be the recipient of a steady stream of vitriol directed toward the President and his decisions. Facial gestures, and almost slanderous words are used to paint an ugly picture of the Nation's President. Fox News, as you might guess, gives a more positive tableau of the President's efforts. The quest for ratings? I don't know. But your decision might depend on your political affiliation. It is a shame that we, the American people, are not united in this war on the virus. I would hate to be on the front lines in this one.

Joe Biden has not yet chosen a running mate. Many Democrats are encouraging Biden to choose a woman. African Americans are suggesting that that person be African American. Wait a minute. It has already been proven that we all, every human being, came out of Africa over two hundred thousand years ago. By the way, I'm proud of that fact, brother.

Been to your local pharmacy lately? Things have changed there, too. At my age, the prescriptions needed to keep me functioning would fill a shopping cart. Noting that some of these life-prolonging drugs were getting low, a call was placed to my local CVS. A phone robot asked questions and I tapped in the required numbers for my refill and I heard, "I'm sorry. We can't seem to find that order." So, off I go to the store to have the order filled at the pharmacist's counter. Over the winter, in Arizona, numbers of prescriptions had changed. The virus? Maybe.

When I arrived at the CVS parking lot, only one other automobile was in the area. In the past, that lot was always full of cars. Months ago, inside that store, you could purchase groceries, pharmaceuticals, toys, candy and everything else to make life comfortable. Not anymore.

Stepping inside the CVS, me in my mask, the familiar six-foot apart circles in the floor guided me toward the pharmacy desk. I walked up to the refill counter. Closed. Going back to the lines in the floor indicating where customers were supposed to stand at attention, I waited. A masked clerk motioned me forward, and I handed her my empty pill container. It was explained, painfully through my cloth mask, what I had encountered on the phone. "Date of birth?" replied the clerk. My prescription order was taken and I was advised to come in the next day for the refill. Needing some other items, my shopping continued, and I approached the register for check out. No clerk. However, a sign read, "We no longer accept cash. Credit card only." I followed directions on the machine, and then I realized that, in the future, even when and if this disease disappears, greenbacks would be a thing of the past. 19 strikes again.

The virus is still causing strife in the country. "You're in the Doghouse Now" was a song done by Brenda Lee in the early 1990's. Lee's lyrics did not make reference to the shut-ins and the sheltering-in-place imposed on us by government officials. But, the title of Brenda's song does seem to have relevance now. When the virus hit months ago, Dr. Anthony Fauci and Dr. Deborah Birx, two respected medical scientists, advised President Trump that Americans should quarantine themselves and stay at home…in the doghouse. Well, not really. But, let's admit that, after months in a closed environment, there is a similarity to the doghouse. Think of the six-foot rule. That's the length of our chain. The masks? Those are our muzzles. Huh? Sure. Try to break out of those restraints. See what happens.

Our grocery stores place signs at their doors reading, "If you are not wearing a mask, please do not come into our store." How about the young mother/hair salon owner in Dallas, Texas? She needed to open her shop in order to earn a living and pay bills. A local judge had the woman arrested, and she was sentenced to seven days in jail. Why was she sentenced to jail? Oh, no, not for breaking a law. She was sentenced to jail because she refused to apologize to the judge for breaking the law. She's now in the doghouse… with you and me. It might just be time to break our chains and show our teeth.

The Chinese are still being accused of a cover up of information relating to the starting point and spread of the COVID-19 virus. Some legislators are calling for reparations. That will, of course, lead nowhere. Democrats are advocating that the government should award every American $1,000 a month to help pay bills. If that were to take place, our country might never recover, and work ethic, something which used to be truly American, would be lost. In Venezuela, two former American special forces men were captured in their attempt to do harm to the Venezuelan President, Maduro. This is something the U.S. does not need…at any time.

Time is moving on. However, the warm weather we were hoping for, the climate change which might have helped kill the virus, is not coming. Snow in the upstate New York area is forecast for Mother's Day.

COVID-19 and its effects on the world's economies cannot be understated. It has already been mentioned that tourism, one of Europe's biggest contributors to the welfare of those nations, is at its lowest point in decades. In the United States, over thirty million people are out of work and are applying for unemployment compensation. Not since the last years of the Great Depression have so many Americans been questioning how they will make ends meet and survive the crisis. In my own community of Saratoga Springs, 19 has raised havoc.

Saratoga has been growing and prospering by leaps and bounds during the last forty years. A bedroom community to the Capital of New York State, Albany, a stable housing market, a rural setting, good schools and recreation offerings have been a Mecca to those in New York City and other large metropolitan communities seeking change. Saratoga is known for its mineral springs, thoroughbred racing, a well-known performing arts center, its city and state parks, and the home of Skidmore and Empire State Colleges. The city has a casino, and its many restaurants sport three and four stars. Condominiums and prestigious hotels attract outsiders from all over the country. Then, out of nowhere, like some giant meteorite striking the Earth, a silent, invisible killer arrived on the scene.

The Saratoga Performing Arts Center, SPAC, has just cancelled its summer performances. The Saratoga Jazz Festival, an event which has drawn thousands to the city each summer for forty-two years has been cancelled. The DMB, Dave Mathews Band and other high-end offerings has been postponed until 2021. The big exclusive hotels which housed concert goers in the past are now empty. Hotel parking lots are desert like in the absence of any sign of human interest. The Saratoga County Fair, an event which drew thousands from all over the state has cancelled its opening for the first time since the Civil War. The city's residents are wondering whether the past will ever return.

Yesterday, the Governor of Texas, Greg Abbott, ordered the release of the Dallas hair salon owner who had been jailed for opening her shop. Uber, the transportation company, is now laying off many of its drivers; no one is venturing out and going to airports. Governor Cuomo is now coming under fire for his ordering nursing home patients to remain sequestered instead of taking them to hospital area such as the Javits Center and the Hospital Ship, Comfort. And, the blame game goes on in the Halls of Congress. Instead of a united front, Democrats and Republicans trade barbs. *Plus ca change, plus c'est la meme chose.* I think that means something like, "I told you so." Maybe not.

Let's continue our chronicle by re-emphasizing what has already been said about trends. Since the invasion of this 19 thing, shopping has changed. Yes, throughout the United States, efforts are now being made in at least ten states to open for business in a partial and safe way. Let it be said that some businesses are doing well, perhaps even better, because service has adapted to the crisis.

At our home, nature is being enjoyed every day. My wife and I feed the wild animals in a variety of ways, and that does attract our feathered friends, squirrels, chipmunks and other four-legged creatures. We have set up a hummingbird station, bird feeders, and we slice up carrots for the wild rabbits in the area. Our feeders remain full for only several days, and then, it's a trip to the wild-bird feed store. Or, it used to be. In the past, I would drive the eight-mile round trip to the mall, get out of my car, go into the store and state my business. Since the shut-down, shopping for bird seed has changed, too.

Yesterday, I made a call to my bird food supplier and asked for procedures now followed. My clerk at the other end of the line advised me that orders were taken over the phone, payment by credit card would be taken, and for a

$5.00 fee, my order would be dropped at my door. Now, let me see. For a small charge, I would not have to leave my home, drive to and from the mall and have my order delivered to my used, time was saved for watching another rerun of Bosch, and I could remain in quarantine. Not only did I like this new normal, my bird-food dropping by our feathered friends (if the birds do not like my choice of seed, it is thrown to the ground) feed the squirrels and chipmunks at the bottom of the feeders. Works for me.

In other news, the DOJ has just dropped all charges against General Michael Flynn who had been accused of lying to the FBI. It now seems that the deep state agents of that federal crime organization might themselves be brought up on charges of falsely building a case against a civil employee. Will anything come of this? Can we tame the wind? There are some who back the FBI completely, and they are the Speaker of the House, the Minority Leader of the Senate, and the head of the Investigative Committee of the House. I forget their names, but political bias does come to mind.

The winds of change have strange bedfellows. As if COVID-19 needed allies in its onslaught against human beings, we are getting close to hurricane season. This is not something to look forward to, and Americans living in the Southeast have already suffered through tornadoes earlier this year. Here in the Northeast, we are experiencing a cold spell, and last night, a light dusting of snow covered plants and lawns. Is Mother Nature angry at the world? Hey, I'm feeding birds here!

Among other things joining the list of cancellations due to the virus is the postponement of the Miss America Beauty

Pageant. As if to counter this cancelled event, the NFL has decided to play its entire season beginning this fall. Whether any spectators will again fill stadiums has yet to be decided. Cameras which used to pan around seated fans will now perhaps be seeing just an array of multi-colored face masks. "Hey, look at that one!"

A lot of appreciative comments and military fly-overs have taken place on behalf of our first responders and health-care personnel for their tireless dedication to work and duty. We tend to forget some others whose job is perhaps just as essential—the trash collectors. Without those workers, tons and tons of garbage would line our streets and attract other things including disease.

Another member of the President's staff has tested positive for the disease I call 19. It is rumored that others in the White House might be axiomatically spreading the virus. Our President is still refusing to wear a mask, but he and others are being tested daily. Be safe, wash your hands… Dry skin, anyone?

MAY 10, 2020

Whether or not the 19 thing is causing Americans to forget that we are in a battle together is confusing. What is true is this: racism on any side of the color barrier, is intolerable. It is with regret that this next report is made. It is sickening, but things do happen here and abroad.

In February of this year in Glynn County Georgia, a young African/American male was allegedly jogging. The young man was 25 years old. From reports gathered later, and with the aid of a film made with a hand-held phone, two white males, a father and son, pulled alongside the jogger, and a dispute occurred. The jogger was shot and killed. Ten weeks later, thanks to someone turning over the filming of the incident, the father and son were taken into custody and held without bail. What has been taking place lately is a continuation of the hatred of American against American.

MSNBC, in a televised report yesterday, held a panel discussion of six journalists, five black and one white participants. A unanimous opinion was formulated; racism has only one color. As the discussion continued, America's love of the 2nd Amendment and the President's approval of that amendment was challenged. The discussing turned into a political lambasting of the White House and its policies.

As once stated before, weekends sometimes show a halt in the basic news, but the Georgia incident held sway for the remainder of the two-day hiatus. But, it, the penchant for heralding poor race relations was not over.

Last Friday afternoon, an African/American young woman was about to enter a Family Dollar Store in Michigan. A security guard at the store told the young woman that she had to wear a mask if she wanted to enter the store. Distraught, the young woman went home, and returned to the store with her adult son and her husband. She then calmly walked up to the security guard and shot him in the back of the head. All three of the black Americans are now being held by the police. The security guard? White or black? I refuse to go there because the implication is too sickening, too utterly devoid of sense to continue. If such things took place in battle, every one of the combatants would be shot. Enough!

News from the World Health Organization reports that we Americans have a long way to go before we will see a break in the effects of the virus or see any form of a vaccine. In the Northeast, Americans are experiencing a cold spell, and overnight, Vermont had four inches of snow. Americans continue to question the stay-at-home and business closing edicts. Maybe rightfully so. In a search of American deaths by natural causes in 2019, over two million people die each year. Are we making too much of this thing which has invaded the world? Could be.

Any good news? Sure, always. Happy Mothers' Day.

MAY 11, 2020

Mother's Day is over. But, many verbal, floral and written tributes were paid to mothers all over the world. Yesterday, Sunday, was one of the bright spots in our week. Today, we begin another period, and from all indications, the positive feelings of the past holiday will be replaced with the bickering of political opinion.

Dry skin anyone? It is difficult to imagine a time in the past when washing my hands took place so often during a day. Life goes on, and so does business, or at least some businesses. Some states are opening up their enterprises. Restaurants, barber shops and hair salons are attracting customers and telling them that gloves and face masks are part of the establishments. Some eating places are using only fifty percent of their once normal spaces, and the social distancing of tables are used. The number of people at each table is limited, too.

Airline companies are parking thousands of their planes on vacated runways in Arizona and in Nevada. Delta is suspending flights to ten cities until next September. Remember seeing bicycle stands along the street where those vehicles could be rented by using a credit card? Those stations now remain empty. I wonder where they parked those bikes. Alongside the airplanes?

In California, Elon Musk, the maker of the electric car, Tesla, has threatened the state by promising to move his industry to Texas. The county in the Golden State where Musk has his main plant refuses to allow the automaker to open his plant during the shutdown. Could politics play a role here, too? Nah! Across the United States, there is a drastic drop in car sales. However, one travel expert does see hope and predicts that Americans will be taking summer road trips instead of getting on airplanes. The travel agent thinks that Americans will fall in love with the road again and take weekend trips with the family.

At the White House, two staffers have tested positive for 19. MSNBC predicts that the entire Trump team will or already has fallen victim to the virus and lessen the effectiveness of the team's effort. Could they, the news media, be wishing that? Nonsense. Dr. Anthony Fauci, and member of the President's team, has self-quarantined himself before his testimony tomorrow at the Senate Committee Hearing on the progress of the WH's team. Will members of the opposition criticize Fauci's efforts or the President's plan? Flip a coin.

The economy? Twenty point five million Americans are out of work. COVID-19 deaths? Seventy-five thousand Americans have lost their lives to the disease. Where's that summer sun which was supposed to scorch the bug? The race card? The killing of the young black-American jogger in Georgia is a constant subject in the news. The killing of a security guard in Michigan by a young black-American woman has lost its media appeal.

Every American community is now a victim of COVID-19. Every little town and hamlet have a story to tell relating to changes force upon it and its population. Here's a tale about my town. In Saratoga Springs, NY, summer home of the Philadelphia Symphony Orchestra, New York City Ballet, the Saratoga Performing Arts Center and one of the country's premier thoroughbred race tracks, try to imagine the grand hotels build over the past twenty years to accommodate the thousands of music lovers, theater goers and racetrack fans. This morning, while taking care of errands in my car, I drove by one of those magnificent lodging places. An empty parking lot and a darkened interior of one of those fine hotels greeted me. It was as if I had been driving through an abandoned Hollywood movie set which was used to film some science fiction invasion of some creatures from outer space. But it was no movie set. It was the scene of a total shut down of what once was a bustling business. It was the reality of what many Americans are facing in the early months of 2020. I wonder what secret weapon could be developed which would rid us of this terrible scourge. Will Tom Cruise suddenly appear and discover that this alien bug is susceptible to fright; that the masks we now wear will cause the thing to burn itself out because of fear? Or, will it, this terrible enemy, take all of us to come out of hiding, face the opponent and suffer the consequences just as we used to do when we caught a bad cold? I'm going with the latter… maybe tomorrow. What do you want to do, live forever?

On the FBI vs the Attorney General, Bill Barr scene, investigators are now looking into the case of General Michael Flynn who allegedly lied to Vice President Pence regarding a phone call to the Russian Ambassador. In disturbing news, it is being reported that Barak Obama, in his last days in office, knew of the FBI's attempts to implicate Flynn in wrongdoing. Last week, charges against Flynn were dropped, and rumor has it that the former National Security Director might be rehired by President Trump. Nothing, however, will erase the legal debt the thirty-year plus Army veteran has suffered.

Today, in the Senate, Dr. Anthony Fauci will testify via television hookups. Liberal journalists and Democrats in Congress are hoping that Fauci will question publicly the President's decision making on the fight against the virus and his ideas on reopening the economy. Media personnel such as Bill Maher are openly hoping that those decisions will put the country into recession so as to improve the chances for a Democrat to take over the country in the November elections.

It is also rumored that China and the United States are in a race to develop an effective vaccine against the virus, and this race is much like that conducted for the race to the moon in the 1960's. In other news, veterans' homes in New Jersey are showing a high death rate for the virus. Seventy-one veterans died in those homes in March. In Virginia, violent criminals are being released for fear that they will test positive for the virus while in prison. So much for recidivism.

MAY 13, 2020

More than several things took place in Washington yesterday. At the White House President's Briefing on the COVID-19 virus, a young female journalist from ABC News spoke up and asked the President, "Why is there such a difference in those testing positive in Korea as compared to the United States? Why are you putting so much emphasis on the amount of coronavirus testing going on in the United States?" At no time did the young woman address Trump as 'Mr. President.' The President's response was, "The United States is doing far better testing than any other country. Why don't you ask China?" Almost immediately, MSNBC anchors called the President a racist because the woman who asked the President a question was an Asian/American. Political affiliation still plays is divisive role in the country… doesn't it.

Yesterday also saw a remote-TV broadcast of a Senate Hearing with members of the President's Task Force on the virus. Dr. Anthony Fauci, CDC Director, Dr. Redfield, Admiral Giroir and Stephen Hahn took questions from the Senate Committee on Reopening the Economy. The following summary of that hearing is given here.

No mention of the names of Senators taking part in the

discussion will be given. Nor will any political designation of those asking questions be mentioned. Make your own decision as to whether the Hearing was partisan of biased. After all the four medical-team members of the President's Task Force gave a five-minute overview of their work, Senators were given five minutes each to ask questions.

The first Senator to speak immediately criticized the President's handling of the pandemic forgetting that by doing so, the entire team receiving the questions were targets of the statement. A question was asked, "Does the model of what is taking place at the White House (several WH staff have tested positive for the virus) serve as a model to other places of work as to how to conduct themselves?" Another Senator asked, "Are the PPE rules in the WH essential for other places?" Someone asked Dr. Fauci, "Your plan was shelved by the administration. How do you feel about that?" Another interlocutor producing plants throughout the United States. Still another mentioned that the fishing industry was having the same problems with the work stoppages going on in the country. One Senator stated that South Korea seemed to be ahead of the U.S. and flattening out the curve of those testing positive and dying. In general, those who watched the hearing might have concluded that partisan politics is still very strong in the Senate. Instead of a united front against the virus, those in Congress are still very much divided.

A genuine concern for whether or not to open the economy was expressed. The fear of a second wave of infections was on the minds of most Senators. Immunity of those who had contracted the disease and recovered was discussed. The question of whether or not a vaccine might be quickly developed came up. The prognosis was not good. However, it was brought out by one of the President's team members that eight different vaccines throughout the world are now being tested.

As evidence of the divisiveness in the media, I made a comparison of two different news media, MSNBC's Joe Scarborough and Mika Brzenzinski vs Fox News' Steve Doocy, Brian Kilmeade and Ainsley Earhardt. Remember the young Asian/American journalist at the WH Briefing and her question about the President's emphasis on testing? MSNBC personnel called the President a racist and a person who is against women. Fox News questioned the journalist and her question as being bias. Make your own decision.

Good news? The Disney Corporation is opening some of its theme parks for the summer. Mickey will be happy.

Is this strange, alien virus causing mental stress and strain throughout the country? It does seem that way. Yesterday, a radio news broadcast reported that some high school girls were concerned about their rights under the Nation's Title IX proposal that females should be able to compete and take part in athletic events. The girls in question stated that they had the right to take part in and compete in athletic endeavors which pitted girls against girls. No problem! That has been the rule since the 1960's. Not anymore. Boys who had been declared male at birth are now claiming to be girls, and they are claiming transgender designation permits them to compete and win in events formally restricted to girls. Oh, well, boys will be…whatever.

In New York State Governor Andrew Cuomo is refusing to use President Trump's definition of the virus as being the "Chinese virus." Media personnel immediately called the President's use of the term as racist. Cuomo, on the other hand is being lauded for his use of the term, "European virus"; it just seems to be more cosmopolitan. No bias here, is there. As long as such antics take place on the public scene, I am wondering why the actors taking part in TV commercials are not required to wear masks. Aren't we in this thing together?

In the on-going case against General Michael Flynn, a federal judge handling the case which is not yet finished, refuses to drop all charges against the former soldier. We did think that the case was over, but the judge has decided to look into the matter further. So, now, we are faced with another new term—"unmasking". Does it refer to the numerous government officials and FBI agents who built a case against General Flynn? Does it refer to naming those accusers? If so, the unmasking of Flynn's accusers might implicate members of President Obama's administration including the Democrat candidate for president in 2020, Joe Biden. I also question the use of the word, "unmasking" when so many of us are encouraged to cover our faces.

Not exactly knowing the meaning of this new and trendy word, I think that I was unmasked this morning. On my way to Dunkin' Donuts, my face covered, I pulled into the drive-through of the store. One of the clerks said, "Hi, Allen". I had been unmasked. Ah, but there is one person who is well aware of the word's meaning, and that is Michael Flynn. This man, a thirty-plus year veteran of service to his country, has lost his home and much more in defense of a charge of perjury, and he could be facing a jail term. Will Flynn's accusers suffer the consequences of what might have been false accusations? Do pigs fly?

It would be pointless and most assuredly fruitless to say that 19 has not affected every aspect of American life. Our economy is that which is most often cited as being the hardest hit by the disease. Wage earners do not get paid if they cannot work…unless, of course, a federal payroll relief package is approved. Hospitals and the pressures put upon them are also mentioned as being on the front lines of the battle, and industries such as the airlines and meat processing plants have been given attention. Now, all of a sudden, as if it is the next domino to topple, the Nation's public schools and universities are coming under scrutiny.

Will our schools reopen after being closed the rest of the 2019-2020 academic year? If an opening does occur, what will classrooms, busing of students, cafeterias and extracurricular activities look like? Will fall sports be played with large crowds of spectators looking on and rooting for the home team? We shall see. Or will we? At this very moment, local, state and federal planners are discussing the restraints under which schools must work.

Early concerns have already been raised and voiced here and abroad as to how schools might work. Teaching staff might have to wear masks and visors. The use of PPE's has been suggested. Hand sanitizers at every classroom door have been mentioned. And, don't forget, *messieurs et dames,* building custodial staff will play an important part in making sure all surfaces in their buildings are safe.

Disinfectant gel dispensers will probably be part of school hallways and student restrooms. Desks in classrooms and in auditoriums will be spaced the required six feet apart. One-day-a-week sessions might occur. Fifteen students per room has been proposed. And, by the way, that might improve classroom discipline unrelated to the virus. Thermal scanners at the entrance to each school building might be used. But, here's the rub. With every one of the above proposals, teaching time and learning opportunities will be diminished because of the necessity to remain safe. Both the quality and quantity of education in our schools will come into question no matter what we employ as shields against the enemy.

Oh, there is at least one more issue facing parents. If you are either a single working parent or a two-parent wage earner with young pre-school children, you will be faced with a dilemma; how will your young children and babies be treated? Will day-care centers and baby sitters be trained and able to keep young children who put everything imaginable in their mouths? Babies need to be held. They might be afraid of someone wearing a multi-colored mask. Babies need to see a smile on the face of those feeding them from a bottle. How are those children delivered to the door of the child-care center? How are they returned to the parent or to someone who is not their parent? Such things are important to Americans with young children…aren't they?

It has just come to light that a COVID-19 related

virus is now affecting young children under the age of five. Day-care center providers are now faced with another weapon used against them. In the end analysis, with all the difference of opinion coming from the right and the left, from conservative and liberal voices, will politics once again stir the waters of discontent so that children suffer? Hopefully, Americans will focus on the lives of those who represent the future.

Dr. Mark Siegel, a frequent contributor to news media coverage, says that no one method of testing is 100% accurate. He also reported that the southern hemisphere, especially Australia, could show a second wave of infection during their winter season. Let's hope and work for the best.

MAY 16, 2020

At the White House yesterday, the President's Briefing on the coronavirus took place with journalists wearing masks. The President's team of scientists working on the development of an effective vaccine are working in an all-out effort to control the disease, and the term, "Operation Warp Speed" is now being used to designate the intensity of the project. It was reported that the possibility of developing a vaccine is good and that it could come as early as December or by the beginning of 2021. Questions followed the announcement of the around-the-clock work project.

Journalists from the news media were interested in knowing whether everyone, not just those considered essential workers, would have access to the vaccine when developed. Other media specialists asked whether the vaccine would be shared with other countries. Still others wondered whether the vaccine might be shared with China. Answers to those questions were affirmative. The briefing showed almost all attendees wearing masks. President Trump did not wear a face covering.

Across the Nation, protests continue to mount up against the stay-at-home policy set by many states. In Wisconsin, a full opening of a bar took place, and most of the bar's customers did not wear masks. More and more Americans are questioning the shutdown which has disrupted work possibilities and closed businesses. Acts of civil disobedience are becoming familiar in reference to laws forbidding gatherings outside the home. Some Americans are wondering how long they can be restricted to their homes when faced with mortgage payments, monthly rents coming due and the purchase of groceries. Unemployment benefits sometimes do not cover monthly bills. Some people are now refusing to wear face coverings, and some of the available masks come with a hole in them allowing room for a straw.

It is hard to imagine that Americans can tolerate more divisiveness in the country coming from many sides of the society. The strife going on in Congress between the Senate and the House of Representatives is paralleled by differences in the media. News coverage of the same story is different depending whether you are for or against the person who won the 2016 presidential election. Reflecting that difference of opinion is the recent 3 trillion-dollar stimulus package just passed by the House. More about that later.

The House of Representatives just passed what it calls, "The Heroes Act". The term was perhaps chosen to draw the interest and appreciation of first responders, health-care workers and what Andrew Cuomo calls, 'essential workers'. This latest relief stimulus package carries a price tag of over three trillion dollars. In its eighteen-hundred-page document, billions of dollars have been allocated to pay off the debts certain American cities have run up over the last two decades. Millions of dollars are supposed to go to undocumented/illegal aliens, and more money will go to the marijuana industry. Those in the Senate are asking why so much money has been designated to areas which have nothing to do with the damage the COVID-19 has caused, and the prognosis of the bill's passing the Senate are not good. One Senator said that instead of sending the bill to the Senate for passage, Nancy Pelosi, the bill's sponsor, should send the package to Santa Clause.

The J.C. Penney Company is now filing for bankruptcy. It will probably join other small businesses which cannot survive because of the lockdown. However, some business are closing their doors to off-the street customers and reverting to on-line ordering. No face masks needed! Let me cite a recent personal on-line shopping incident which is saving some enterprises.

Every spring, *Madame* Remaley takes charge of our outdoor floral arrangements. She usually goes to the neighborhood garden nursery, chooses live flowers in hanging baskets and pays a few hundred dollars for her home-beatification projects. Not this year. The virus, social distancing, shelter-in-place, face-covering edicts have forced change. Thinking that shopping for live plants might take more time and effort than it's worth, (all the above plus transportation of self and product), she decided to see what might be available in artificial flowers and hanging baskets. Amazon came to the rescue. Not only did my wife find some beautiful arrangements, the cost of her outdoor project was cut in half. The plastic/synthetic flowers arrive in the next few days, and with them, an added bonus—no weekly watering. On-line shopping is becoming popular.

Another phenomenon just came to my attention. Throughout the United States, dog pounds and kennels are running low on puppies. The six-foot rule, social distancing and sheltering-in-place restrictions have caused Americans to develop a new disease—'skin hunger'. Huh? Yes, the expression, 'skin hunger' refers to the fact that we cannot any longer get close to one another. We cannot shake hands or hug anyone. The inability of not being able to reach out to someone and express our admiration, love and appreciation to another human being has left a desire to return to a skin-on-skin token of affection.

In the United States at the present moment, dogs and other pets have become important. Americans are scooping up pets, and these little creatures offer unconditional love to their owners. Hugging has been reborn. Even for the widow or widower, the single parent or elderly shut-in, a stuffed animal might do the trick. We all need someone or something to love during this time of plague.

COVID-19 has led to multiple problems for those at the university level of education. A female student at Yale University recently found herself at home because classes had been suspended during the shutdown. However, her clothes were left in her leased apartment at school. Her lease runs out at the endo of May, and she has been asked to sign another lease for the coming school year, 2020-2021…if it ever comes. Sometimes, things do not seem to get easier as we go along in life…do they.

The weekend is over. Reruns of the past week's events had flooded the networks Saturday and Sunday, and there were reports of growing unrest over the lockdown and its restrictions. In New York State, protests took place in Albany concerning Governor Cuomo's hesitancy to allow businesses to open. New Yorkers and others across America are now beginning to question why small shops, gyms and barber shops are forced to fail, and they are upset over responses to their questions. In one of Governor Cuomo's daily press conferences held last week, one onlooker asked the governor why she was not allowed to work. Cuomo replied, "You want to go to work? Get a job as an essential worker." That king-like response did not sit well with those who have been out of work these last three months.

Ever wonder what happened to the 2019-2020 protests by Chinese students in Hong Kong? Those protests started in the fall of 2019, when the Chinese government passed the 'Fugitive Offenders' Amendment. That bill allowed the mainland government of China to extradite criminal suspects to territories not working with Hong Kong legislature. Knowing that some of the 'criminal suspects' were dissident students, riots broke out, and thousands of students flooded the streets. Pictures of those acts of civil disobedience show something interesting. Photos and films show both rioters and police wearing N95 masks and PPE's. In some of the pictures, rioters are carrying umbrellas in order to prevent being showered with a spray coming from water trucks. Ever wonder what might have been in that liquid spray? Coincidences or not, the protests ceased in late December 2019, and early 2020, and coincided with the outbreak of COVID-19. Hum?

Such unsubstantiated information causes paranoia to set in. A few months ago, my Hamilton wristwatch stopped keeping time. When a jeweler told me that a repair would cost several hundred dollars, I went to Wal-Mart. For $14.00, I bought a new watch…made in China. A few days ago, my left wrist began to give me pain. Oh, OK, I know that no radio-active materials were used in the manufacturing of a timepiece…don't I. I still wear the watch…most of the time.

Remember the hype coming out of some media about the FBI's attempt to implicate President Trump in various crimes and misdemeanors against the Nation? Not much mention is made of that fruitless effort now. However, as soon as the Attorney General of the United States began an unofficial inquiry into the people involved in unmasking Michael Flynn, attention was diverted from that issue to the firing of Steve Linick, the Inspector General. Linick was allegedly looking into wrongdoings by the Secretary of State, Mike Pompeo who, it is rumored, asked one of his deputies to do some personal work for him and his wife. Collusion, crimes and misdemeanors, improper use of government employees! So, the investigation into

Biden, Comey, Mueller, Clapper et al, was dropped. So was the investigation into the Senators who had used insider trading information to make millions. Yes, Republican and Democrat Senators. Oh, well, bigger fish to fry.

Personal experience, subjecting the self into an account of the daily happenings influenced by a crisis, might not lend itself to good reading. On the other hand, let the reader choose just as the American worker is now contemplating whether or not to return to the workplace. Everyone has a right to read or skip over words on paper.

Today, all across the United States, Americans are asking themselves how long this sheltering-in-place is going to last. They, those who have needs above and beyond the entitled person, the welfare recipient, the receiver of social security payments or elected officials whose pay is guaranteed, are faced with the question of making ends meet. So, here it comes. What would I do if my place of business was vital to my livelihood as well as those I might employ?

As a seventeen-year-old in Marine Corps boot camp, I waited for graduation and a fifteen-day leave before reporting to my first duty station. I returned to my home town, and during my military leave, I worked in the local tannery, a business which later went to some Asian country. The money I earned during those two weeks made my life as a Pfc a little better. After my four-year enlistment as a grunt, my matriculation to university studies began, and

I thought that my four years as a Marine would entitle me to unemployment insurance benefits. Wrong! When it came time for me to request those benefits, a clerk at the Unemployment Bureau told me that since I was going to school full time, my being available for work eliminated me from any entitled benefits. That same day, I began working in a men's clothing store and continued to do so for the next four years and paid for my own college education. And, yes, my paycheck had a deduction for unemployment insurance taxes. But something else happened. I developed a work ethic which has remained with me for over fifty years. And, that allows me to know what other Americans are feeling. They want to get back to work and feel…essential.

Today, after three months of shut down, Americans are protesting about remaining at home, sheltering-in-place and wondering whether there will be any future. That sense of discontent is percolating and is about to boil over. Americans have been told that, if they exercise their right to work too soon, if they return to what they believed to be normal, they might die. Americans also know that the advice they have been given comes from salaried employees like those in Congress, like those other elected officials who have not yet seen the stress of being out of work. Two hundred years ago, the expression, "Taxation without representation" defined a reason for going to war. It might be time to allow Americans to return to the workplace and do so safely.

In other news, Oxford University is developing a vaccine against the virus, and if it is successful, that vaccine will be available in September of this year and shared with the other nations in the world. In the 3 trillion-dollar relief package proposed by the House of Representatives, no part of the bill would protect employers from being sued by employees who might contract 19 while in the workplace. In this day and time, such a thing would most assuredly occur, and some business owners might be hesitant to hire their help. The Senate has proposed that business owners be protected from lawsuits, and unless that idea is incorporated into future relief plans, passage of such a thing is unsure.

On Fox News this morning, one of the hosts said, "The lockdown is over because the American people say that it is over." My guess is that civil disobedience will grow in direct proportion to the demand to remain in shut down. Elon Musk recently said, "Take the red pill!" I wonder what he meant by that. I'll ask MSNBC and CNN. They'll tell me.

MAY 20, 2020

Why am I taking the time to write this book? I could be playing pickle ball. Wait! Courts are closed; we are in a pandemic. The same happenings and decision making coming from elected officials and scientific and medical personnel could be researched years from now on Wikileaks. My guess is that most facts of the day will have been changed by revisionists. Time does that to people who were not there at the moment of crisis. But, the little mundane stories of what the average American is experiencing during this trying time should be told in the present tense and remembered in the future. The roadblocks and hurdles placed in our path by either elected officials or select members of the medical profession must be told.

Both successes and failures should be documented. Their efforts and mistakes should be pointed out. Remember the female physician giving the public advice on how to conduct themselves in public in an effort to avoid contagion? She explained that social distancing and sheltering-in-place were essential, and that washing one's hands and not touching the face or eyes should be done often. And then, to help her turn the page in her notes, she wet her finger with her tongue and turned the page to give us more information.

Writing things down might prevent a repetition of wrong decision making and provide a road map of how to navigate through obstacles in the future. Ah, yes, the machinations of Congress, the biases of the media and the political partisan behavior of elected officials needs to be outlined as well. Contrasting the past with what we hope will not occur in the future might save time, money and lives.

In New York State, Governor Cuomo has come under fire for his decision to place those who tested positive in nursing homes where the spark of the virus caused a forest fire of contagion and death. Why those who were infected were not placed in the government-provided hospital constructed in the Javits Center or on board the USS Comfort in New York harbor is still a mystery. Things like that could be avoided in the future…if they are recorded and brought to light by the media. Could the decision to place ill people in nursing homes instead of places offered by Washington by political. Of course not.

The State of Arizona opened places of business today. Three months ago, when my wife and I were there, a dark, somber atmosphere had descended upon the Valley of the Sun. Now, when that sun is raising the temperature to 95 and above, perhaps the sun's rays will scorch and burn up some of the virus. Judging from films shown at Phoenix restaurants, people are once again moving about in relative and happier moods. Let's hope that a resurgence of 19 does not dispel the warmth now felt.

The Secretary of State, Mike Pompeo, has been criticized for his firing of the Inspector General, and Obama appointee who was conducting an investigation into the Secretary's alleged use of an associate to walk the Secretary's dog.

Collusion! This allegation comes at the exact time when the Attorney General, Bill Barr, is investigating the unmasking of Michael Flynn by members of the past administration and the FBI. Coincidence! Where's Adam Schiff?

Bumper tables! What? Yes, one east coast beach-side bar has recently equipped its tables with wraparound rubber tires. The tables are on wheels and they are three-foot-wide on each side of the table's occupant thus assuring the proper six-foot distancing. Another innovation during the crisis comes into play. My guess that each occupant of such a table would not hesitate answering, "May I get you another?"

"Why, you fat slut!" Please forgive me for using such a misogynistic and bully-like expression. Imagine anyone, let alone a male member of Congress, using such a terminology to describe the physiognomy of a fellow female colleague. Could you imagine the user, the speaker of such an unflattering terminology being able to continue to serve in the legislative branch of government? Me, either. No, the vulgar use of such a term did not come from Donald J. Trump. However, a similar put-down did come from one member of Congress—a woman. We will get to that.

Yesterday, the President announced that he had been taking a limited dosage of the anti-malarial drug, hdroxychloroguine, as a prophylactic against COVID-19. Many medical scientists and physicians have expressed reservations about the drug. But, in some cases, people who have used it stated that the symptoms of the disease of those contaminated were minimal, and a few others have said that the taking of the drug cured them completely. Scientific testing of the drug is still inconclusive. However, the drug has been in use in the United States for two decades. The American President who does not yet wear a mask seems to be looking for a fast and effective substitute for a vaccine.

Media spokespersons have criticized the President for his faulty and dangerous precedent setting. They have accused the President of offering false hopes to the American people, and some reporter/journalists have accused him of killing Americans. So much, come close to that used by the Speaker of the House, Nancy Pelosi, the same woman who, at the end of the President's State of the Union Address in January, tore to shreds a copy of the official document. Yesterday, when told of the President's using the hydroxychloroquine, Pelosi said that taking the drug was dangerous and that "he is so morbidly obese." Was our Speaker admonished by anyone in the media or by any of her liberal colleagues? Do you see a flying armada of porcine-like animals?

Folks, we have come to a new low in our civility toward others. Unfortunately, such a descent into foulness comes when we are in the middle of a pandemic. It comes when we have lost ninety thousand Americans to the disease. Whether you are Democrat or Republican, we deserve better from members of Congress.

Elsewhere in the news, Delta Airlines is adding flights on major routes. Royal Caribbean Cruise Lines is eliminating its famous buffet. Nineteen million dollars has been given to Farm Aid which will help food delivery to markets. Professional sports are contemplating a fall season without spectators. One former professional football player, when asked whether fans would be needed, responded, "In summer camp, no one is there. In scrimmages, no one attends. We'll make do." Let's hope all of us do.

MAY 22, 2020

How has the COVID-19 affected visits to your family physicians? Yesterday, I had an appointment with my ophthalmologist in a check for how my cataracts were doing. Good idea to keep an eye on them. Knowing that restrictions would be imposed on those wishing to see their doctors (I live in New York State), a call was made to the doctor's office in order to be brought up to date on how to conduct myself and get the new mitigation advice we must follow. The phone receptionist informed me that masks were de rigueur and that once I had arrived at the office, I would have to make a call, report that I had arrived and follow instructions. Worse than checking into TSA at the airport. I was told that someone would come out into the parking lot, take my temperature, ask whether I was suffering from headaches, coughs, nausea, sore throat or malaria. I was hoping that the temperature screening would take place above the belt.

At the appointed time, I pulled into the doctor's parking lot, made the required call, and the pre-appointment interview took place over the phone. Thank goodness, no temperature taking took place. You never know. I was then asked to come into the office waiting room. Inside, we traded medical cards, and I was officially checked in. Other patients were already seated…six-feet apart, and some chairs were turned toward the walls, and very efficiently spaced adhering to prescribed protocol. Both waiting patients and desk personnel were wearing masks. Mine was a patriotic American-flag rendition. I took a seat at one of the chairs facing inward. Better to keep an eye on things. After all, I was at an ophthalmologist's office. While waiting my turn to see the doctor, I coughed, not on purpose, of course, but just to clear my throat. Those around me changed chairs and the six-foot rule became the ten-foot rule.

Soon, I was conducted into the inner sanctum of the examining room and verbally screened by a mask-wearing young attendant. My eye pressures were taken and recorded, visual fields taken and other tests which were probably eye-related were conducted. My eyes were dilated, and I waited for Dr. Christopher Zieker to give me news on how my cataracts looked.

Dr. Zieker is a young, down-to-earth practicing ophthalmologist. He is a red, white and blue advocate of protecting the American way of life, and on past occasions, has indicated that he is proud of those who served their country in uniform. I always make sure I wear some USMC gear to his office. Makes me feel good, too. When the doctor came into the examination room, we exchanged greetings, and he apologized for not shaking hands. We both understood. You know, cameras and snitching. An overview of the tests performed on me before his arrival into the room was given. We exchanged opinions about the present state of life with the virus, and then he brought me up to date on the almost-daily changes concerning mitigation. I was told that a study had come out pertaining to table tops and other surfaces which previously had been considered dangerous. No longer. Flat surfaces are no longer considered dangerous for contagion. Must make a lot of supermarket checkout clerks happy. They have been wiping down those surfaces after every customer passes through. My guess is that those surfaces are clean enough to serve jello on. As the examination continued, I was told that something was going on in my right eye that needed further examination. According to the doctor, what was found might have been a false positive, and that I should return to the doctor's office in ten days. The doctor also explained that things were moving along very well, and that on my next appointment, masks might not be required. He also said that he was happy because now, in a more opened atmosphere, he could continue to perform operations on those who had been waiting on operation-room procedures. Are things opening up…in New York State?

Update on the growing trend of changing opinions about the virus and its affects takes place daily. Scientists, medical personnel, politicians and the media come up with perfect descriptions about how we should look at the disease. The following day, those opinions are shot down, and a new set of directives are paraded before the public. Americans sit back and say, "Well, they must know what they are doing." Not anymore. One of the latest discoveries has to do with how one contracted the disease in the past. We were advised to wear gloves because everything we touched was contaminated. Supermarket check-out clerks are asked to wipe down their check-out surfaces after every customer has paid and left the area. Once that chore is completed, the clerk motions to the next customer to begin laying out his groceries. Those check-out surfaces have to be the cleanest places in the world. Now, we are learning that viruses do not spread easily on smooth surfaces. Yesterday, check-out clerks were still wiping down their automatic check-out belts. Adherence to directives. Isn't it wonderful?

In other changes, a number of physicians are stating that sheltering-in-place should remain in force. A similar number of medical personnel are advocating that we end the shut down and encourage a full opening of business. This tug of war, a playground and amusement-park event, is being governed by what political party you support. If a suggestion comes from Washington, certain media and other professional talking heads object, and pull in an opposite direction. Makes for great entertainment, and it —that never-ending Kabuki theater goes on forever. Must be political.

Americans are well into the second month of the pandemic, and in spite of many state and federal efforts to rid ourselves of this deadly scourge, there is still a great amount of hatred and bias which is holding the country hostage. We are unable to join hands (oops, *faux pas*) and form a united front in this battle against 19. A Trump-hating media controlled by political affiliation makes cowards of us all; we are all too hesitant to tolerate the ideas of others. There is now even talk about a second impeachment investigation. Had it not been for the first three-month long waste of time, Washington might have had its ey23es on things going on in a city in China. Ah, but grudges are hard things to drop.

Today, on my one-day-a-week supermarket visit, watching check-out clerks mindlessly wiping down counters, I happened to pass by the ubiquitous slander and scandal magazines. On the front page of one of those tabloids, a big ad read, "Lose thirty pounds before Memorial Day". I almost went for it, but since today is May 23, I thought my chances of dropping thirty pounds before Memorial Day were pretty slim. The virus has even slowed delivery of the rumor-mill pages. Before we move on to another day, this might be the time to review some of the wording used to disguise inability to define the bug.

New Normal Expressions for 19

Skin hunger   contagion   lockdown

Remdesivir   Wusan   hydroxychloroquine

Chloroquine   CDC   WHO

Asymptomatic   Contact tracing   flattening the curve

Hospital ships   pestilence   Operation Warp Speed

COVID-19   pandemic   remote hearing

Ventilators   respirators   curb-side-pickup

Unmasking   SCOTUS   POTUS

Six-foot rule   PPE's   shelter-in-place

PSP   resurgence   social distancing

Vaccine   collusion   on-line-shopping

Antibodies   testing positive   quarantine fatigue

Relief package   USS Mercy   Exculpatory evidence

USS Comfort   N95 masks   herd immunity

The apex   mitigation   screening

Shut down   opening up   flare up

—Hey, Allen, you missed a couple!

—Well, fill em' in. You're a big girl now.

MAY 24, 2020

Even in this atmosphere of plague, there is still evidence that the concept of haves and have nots is working its way through the thoughts of some Americans. Lori Laughlin, a T.V. personality, and her husband were recently charged with fraud for illegally buying their daughter's way into USC. For months, the daughter's millionaire parents fought the courts but finally pled guilty to the crime. Both the father to five, the ubiquitous double standard in treatment of men and women. I do wonder whether both husband and wife will plead for mercy claiming the probable chance of contracting the virus while in prison. Might depend on alumni.

The governors of certain blue states are adamant about not opening up businesses. Might it have to do with bolstering the economy too soon? It does seem that, if the President proposes something, just the opposite will be advocated by the opposition. Some reluctant governors are saying that they cannot open up their states until a vaccine is developed. Some medical scientists say that there might never be a vaccine. In such a scenario, the United States could turn into another Venezuela. That divisiveness has filtered its way down to small communities and into families.

Recently, *Madame* passed by one or our former neighbors on a walk. My wife said hello to the woman who was wearing a mask, and when asked how she was doing, the woman said, "Well, not bad. I'm saving lives." My wife needed an explanation, and the woman continued, "My brother is a Trump supporter, and he doesn't wear a mask. I don't see much of him anymore, and I am saving lives by not seeing anyone who does not follow the guidelines." My wife continued her walk, readjusted her mask and said nothing about the woman's brother who works three jobs to put his son through school. One of those jobs took place at the thoroughbred racetrack, an operation which will not take place this year.

Religious dogma is also playing a role in dividing us. Two days ago, a Syrian-born man drove his automobile into the Naval Air Station in Corpus Christi, Texas and shot a police guard. The shooter, later identified as an Islamic terrorist was killed. His accomplice is being sought but not yet found. Oh well, terrorists will be terrorist.

Some airlines are flying again, but the middle seats are blocked off. TSA has proposed new changes to its policies. No temperatures will be taken before boarding. Food must be carried in separate plastic bags and placed in special bins for examination. Hand sanitizer bottles must not exceed 12 oz. All other liquids must not exceed 3.4 oz. Social distancing will take place in the TSA lines. Facial coverings will be required and pulling them down for person recognition will take place. Anyone remember when flying was fun?

Finally, more members of Congress are working hard to introduce liability insurance for employers who might be sued by their workers who claim they were infected while being required to work. Oh, well.

Memorial Day! God bless the men and women who stormed the beaches, bled in the forests and suffered the heat of the deserts to guarantee freedom of speech, religion and the American way of life.

Over the weekend, President Trump announced that houses of worship should open up immediately. However, he might have gone too far in stating that governors who kept their state' churches closed would deal with him. Saying such things make him look Cuomo-like, and we do not need any more kings. And, being tolerant, whether you are president or governor can lead to undue criticism. Questions have come up as to whether schools will start up again in the fall. Sports taking place during that season of the year have questions to be answered. The summer is already heating up with Americans trying to decide what is right and what is safe.

Hertz Rental Car Company has filed for bankruptcy. Americans who no longer travel do not need to pick up transportation at airports. The FBI has come under more scrutiny for its mishandling of the Michael Flynn case. That political football has been passed around more than a Brady to Gronkowski third and long situation. Once again, politics has raised its ugly head above the crowd. So, what should take place? Should my writing stop and wait for the pickle ball courts to reopen? Let me tell you what I would like to see.

If I had a magic wand, with one sweep, an effective vaccine would be developed which would insure herd immunity and wipe out COVID-19 throughout the world, houses of worship would be filled with appreciative parishioners, more Americans than ever would be at work supporting their families and their communities, restaurants and bars would be filled with customers not wearing masks, women would be flocking to hair salons and men to barber shops, schools would be filled with students happy to see their friends again and not relying on virtual learning, sports venues would be jammed with cheering fans, mass outdoor concerts would ring with the music of the day. Well, you get the idea, and I am sure you could add to the wand's list of hoped-for outcomes. But, realism must be considered.

Let's hope for the best and not give up. I'm not. I will continue to record, document and cite efforts to rid us of the medical and economic disaster. Why not? It's better than watching reruns of SNL. Oh, by the way, do you pray? My religious affiliation is personal, but I tend to go along with Blasé Pascal, a seventeenth-century philosopher and mathematician who said, "If I believe in God and life after death and you do not, and if there is no God, we both lose when we die. However, if there is a God, you still lose and I gain everything, and you go to Hell". I'll hedge my bets. Might be safer.

Let's do some, "What if's". What do we have to lose? What is some scientist working in the 'Warp Speed' team were to come up with a successful vaccine against the virus? What if Democrats and Republicans were to work together on putting the country back to work? What if those in the FBI who might have been illegally vetting Michael Flynn were found guilty and sentenced? What if Nancy Pelosi and Donald Trump were to sponsor a Memorial Day get together for Americans? What if…? Wait! I forgot. We are in shut down. Social distancing must be maintained. Sheltering-in-place must continue. Where's my mask?

Duplicity, that sometimes deceitfulness which lurks just beneath the surface of human endeavors, is now with us. We are witnessing a political divide in the United States, and it hinges on two things: the unending hatred of the American President, Donald J. Trump, and the impending presidential election to take place later this year. In back-room political party meetings, most of which are closed to the public, strategies are outlined as to how decisions will be made concerning what should take place in the Nation. Today, across the country, the government in Washington (Republican) is advocating the opening of businesses. Washington's opponents (Democrats) must do and say the opposite. Stalemate.

Blue states and advocating a stay-at-home policy. Red states are asking that a return to normal take place. Supporters of both sides of the political spectrum are at odds. Governors who have ruled that beaches, gyms, hair salons and barber shops remain closed stick close to the party line. Opponents of such decisions are now openly protesting in the streets and unlawfully opening their places of business. They march carrying placards, American flags, and they voice their wishes via bullhorns in protest. And, it, this turmoil, boils down to two things: you are either a supporter of Joe Biden or Donald Trump. Not much thought is given to corralling the virus. Isn't politics interesting.

Have we mentioned the college football season? Will churches and other places of worship be opening soon? The answers to those questions might depend on the number of people in favor of one or the other. The larger number of those supporting an issue means more votes. In the long run, those watching from the sidelines might be the losers.

Laying blame on others is also something we encounter. Andrew Cuomo, New York State Governor, recently made the decision to place those who tested positive in nursing homes with senior citizens. He chose not to use beds in the USS Comfort or in the Javits Center, facilities provided by a different political affiliation. Many of the elderly in those nursing homes contracted the disease and died. Cuomo's comment on the case was, "You can't blame the state for something the President did." What? Let's go to a more positive example of how some Americans are doing a better job.

An unexpected and very generous act just took place in my community, and it involves my daughter, Janine. Janine is a private day-care provider for children of parents who teach in Saratoga. She works out of her home, and she usually has four to five pre-school children from the same number of families. When schools closed in April of this year, Janine was out of a job and without income; she was ineligible for unemployment insurance. That is when one of the two-teacher families decided to continue paying Janine for having been there when needed. That unselfish and generous showing of support is worthy of mention, and it shows character above and beyond that expected. Some Americans are still on the front lines during the battle.

Yesterday, at Fr. McHenry, the site of the English attack on the American stronghold where Francis Scott Key penned the "Star-Spangled Banner", President Trump laid a wreath to commemorate this Nation's dead. Later, the President did the same at the Tomb of the Unknown Soldier in Washington. Over the past centuries, over 500,000 men and women have given their lives in defense or liberty and independence. While performing his duties in honoring fallen heroes, the President was probably thinking of other things more political.

The Governor of the State of North Carolina is now questioning whether or not to allow full attendance in a pavilion scheduled to host the Republican National Presidential Convention. The governor, a Democrat must first think of the health of Republicans who are supposed to meet in Charlotte in late August of this year. The rope used in the political tug of war is getting stretched to the breaking point. Trump has threatened to take the convention to the State of Florida. Democrats are hoping that the Republicans will chose one of Trump's properties as the venue. Now, wouldn't that provide reasons for criticism! "Trump is using the American voters to fill his coffers as he runs for president." Or, something like that.

The word, "essential" has often come up. Whether to open for business or to continue the shutdown seems to depend on whether or not a worker is 'essential'. One T.V. commentator suggested that, "What is essential is the American people." More and more Americans are going along with that idea. They are enforcing that thought by going to the beaches, getting their hair cut at barber shops, having an appointment at the beauty parlor and sitting at outdoor restaurants…unmasked.

Today at 4:33 P.M. in Florida, America's first shot into space from American soil will take place in a vehicle designed by private citizens. The Space-X capsule on top of an American rocket and manned by two astronauts will head out for the International Space Platform. The two astronauts will join one other already in place and conduct experiments in a zero-atmosphere situation. This launch from Florida will be followed by others on the way to the moon and ultimately, to Mars. Let's hope the virus needs air to survive and none of the stuff is found in outer space.

In the political arena, life goes on. Joe Biden, the Democrats' candidate for President in now blaming Trump for all American deaths from COVID-19. President Trump tweets back that Biden might be a fool. Ah, civility, will it ever return? As long as we remain true believers, probably not.

Over the last weekend and extending into Wednesday, the last full week in May, violence is occurring at an increasing rate across the United States. In Albany, seven shootings took place within the last four days. Two people were wounded, and no suspects were arrested. In Chicago, the number of shootings has risen, and like New York's Capital, no suspects have been rounded up. In Minnesota, a black American was killed by police officers in what has caused a flare up of looting and civil disobedience. Is politics playing a role here or does Eric Hoffer's 1960' "The True Believer" coming to pass?

In Hoffer's book, individuals whose beliefs were unchangeable, steel-like in their adherence to dogma and who saw only one path to life made a name for themselves. Hitler was a true believer. Today, some people say that they are wearing masks because it saves lives. They berate people who break rules and choose not to wear face coverings. The mask wearer, the true believer, sometimes become violent and anger turns into intolerance which causes death. Is it the virus and the stress it causes part of the problem? Your guess.

Another anti-social phenomenon is taking place. In the above paragraphs concerning shootings, no suspects were taken. No snitching took place and in spite of everyone carrying cell phones, no films of the shootings ever came to light. However, in adherence to medical advice, if you are not wearing a face covering, someone, a true believer, will out you by calling the police or warning store owners that the uncovered one is violating the rules. Snitching in that case is acceptable. Those who openly go to the beach or attend religious gatherings are now suspects. If you are seen going into a church, someone will burn it down as was the case recently in Georgia. Who is right here? Could politics be hindering our progress toward unity? Oh, Hell, no. Well, maybe.

Been to the grocery store lately? Of course, you have. At my market, masks are de rigueur. Do some shoppers choose not to wear masks? Certainly. I don't chase them down and yell, "You're killing people." Besides, my voice isn't what it used to be. If I did that, I would be a true believer. I'm not going there. There are too many TB's on the street as it is. Tolerance is such a hard thing to master.

I'm looking forward to this afternoon. At 4:33 P.M. E.T., America's first launch into space from American soil is to take place. I'm betting our astronauts will be wearing masks. They are true believers…the good kind. God bless them. I would not want to be riding that air capsule.

MAY 28, 2020

Brutality in any form, especially when committed by uniformed officers of the law, those first responders so revered in fly overs and clapping of hands, should never be tolerated. Within the last few days, police in Minneapolis arrested a black American, George Floyd, who allegedly broke the law by trying to pass a $20.00 counterfeit bill. Then, for many minutes, one of the arresting officers held Floyd down by putting a knee across Floyd's neck. Floyd died. Four of the arresting officers were immediately fired and no further prosecution has taken place since that time. That's when rioters broke into stores, set them afire and looted the contents of shops nearby. This incident is not over. Police and citizens all over the country will continue to suffer from the fallout of such a dastardly act.

Lawlessness is becoming more prevalent with each day. A woman in a grocery store just this morning spat on a man who was not wearing a mask and going the wrong way down one of the aisles. The woman had to pull her own mask down to commit her disgusting and intolerable act. I am guessing that she believed that she was saving lives by being politically correct—a political correctness in reverse however. Bad cops, bad neighbors. Ah, those First Amendment Rights!

Joe Biden has not yet chosen a running mate, but he is on the campaign trail. In an interview with a black American talk-show host, Biden was asked if he expected support from black American voters. Biden's reply was, "If you have to ask that question, then you ain't black". The next morning, after much criticism, Biden apologized for his off-the-cuff remark. Just between you and me, those going to the ballot box should wear gloves and masks to hide one's skin color. It should not make any difference what ethnicity you profess when you do anything, and that includes voting.

Ah, but the day does show hope. Today, at 4:33 P.M., at Cape Canaveral, Florida, an American space capsule, the Dragon, will lift off and carry two American astronauts into space for the first time in a decade from American soil. For the remainder of the afternoon, I will watch as the two former military pilots, one a Marine, the other Air Force, ready themselves for a one to four-month visit to the International Space Platform high above the Earth. Families of the astronauts watched as the two men, both fathers, waved their goodbyes to wives and children.

While I watched, a very disturbing thought entered my mind, and I struggled with it. Along with the majority of other Americans, I prayed for the safety and the success of the launching knowing that a million things could go wrong. But, the dark thought that others, not so patriotic, not so interested in America's positive values, might wish for less successful results. Those true believers whose ideals and political goals are held to be more important than human life, might tip the scales of right and wrong.

Couldn't happen. At that very moment, word was passed that, because of inclement weather, the liftoff was being shut down. A rescheduling was to take place, Saturday, May 30. May God protect us all.

The virus? That's the least of our problems at the moment. Our biggest threat is not COVID-19. Our biggest threat is rampant and open defiance of the law in the name of racism. The rioting, looting and self-justified mayhem taking place in Minneapolis and in other American cities has taken our sights off of a disease which attacks the body from outside the skin, and it has been replaced with something which takes place in the mind. Yesterday, protesters rioted, looted and burned a police station and other buildings to the ground. In response to the unjustified killing of George Floyd, an alleged user of counterfeit money, civil disobedience took over the streets, bodies and minds of some Americans.

In the above disturbances, no social distancing was adhered to. Yes, masks were used, but not to deter contagion, they were used to prevent identification. The National Guard has been called out to protect firefighters who are now engaged in quelling fires set overnight. So, our number one culprit is not some invisible, silent incurable disease. COVID-19, forget that. As unfortunate as it is to say, it seems that black against white and white against black is the thing that is more dangerous than the virus.

Everyone who has seen the brutal killing of George

Floyd in Minneapolis is sickened by the sight. Protesters and looters practicing their rituals were not using social distancing. Far from it. But they were wearing masks. Those masks were not worn as protection from the virus. They were work so as to not be recognized. Is there any solution to this social disobedience? Who knows? Is there a solution to unbridled racism? Same answer. However, there is a suggestion.

In Minneapolis, there should be an immediate arrest of all police officers who were part of the initial conflict. In the speediest trail in history, all those accused should be tried, and if convicted, an immediate sentence should be carried out. And, the same should occur with those who set fires, looted and ruined public property. Will that end the violence? No, not at all. In some human being, DNA, tradition, hopelessness and social hatred based on one's ethnic, religious or lifestyle will break the peace. But one thing was evident during the protesting: people are not worried about some infection taking place. Many have already proved that getting out in public might be safe. That violent opening up might awaken those who need to get out and get to work. And, now, the $20.00 bill. If the clerk who thought the bill was bogus would have just warned George, given it back to him and go about business…in other words, used tolerance, hum!

Ah, tomorrow, the continuation of the countdown to sending Spacex or Space-X to the International Space Station. Can't wait!

A famous author once said, "This is the best of times and the worst of times." That sums up my thinking on the issues at the moment. Looking back at the killing of George Floyd in Minneapolis four days ago, a progression of events, all of them bad, has taken place. On the first day after the brutality against a black American, we sympathized with the demonstrators. On the second day after the atrocity, we questioned the rioters and looters. On the third day after the nonsensical act, we withdrew in disgust our support for all those involved in the rioting, looting and burning of public property and places of business. On this, the fourth day after the violence committed against a fellow American, we call for an immediate crackdown on the anarchists committing crimes against communities across the United States. Both COVID-19 and George Floyd are forgotten.

The administrations in Minneapolis, Chicago, Atlanta, Cincinnati and other American cities must now be questioned. How is it possible that the mayors, city councils and police departments are able to stand aside and watch vandalism and mayhem take place before their eyes? How is it possible to watch vehicles, shops and buildings be destroyed without any attempt to control the mobs? Is this a political move? Are the governing officials saying that we had it coming? Even the media is reluctant to throw blame on the nihilists involved in what some people call protests. Who had it coming? Americans who lost their jobs because of an incurable virus? Americans who lost their source of income because their place of work went up in smoke? What crap. Black against white, white against black—ridiculous, unnecessary and a waste of time, money, ego, pride…ah, Hell, you add the rest. There are better things to contemplate.

This morning, a local, more rural news media affiliate documented the story of a young mother who had just spent thirty days in hospital, two days in coma with the virus. The woman was released today, and she was awarded with applause and a drive by parade of her friends, of all ethnicities. It was heartwarming. By the way, the recovering victim of the virus was a black American. I thank God that I was able to record something more than the description of an angry group of thugs formed into an unruly mob seeking vengeance for a man whose name the rioters could not recall or spell.

Will the atrocities of the past four days be repeated? With some trepidation, I doubt that some city officials will have either the will or the courage to call an end to the madness. But, as for me, I will not spend the next few hours glued to the T.V. watching the nihilist mentality of the mob. I'm too old, and we do have a more-positive event coming up—the Crew Dragon Space-X launch of our two astronauts who will fly to the International Space Platform. Hell of a lot more interesting and certainly more uplifting.

—Wait! Aren't you going to watch the continuation of looting and burning?

—Are you nuts? That will only take place after curfew under cover of darkness.

OK, let's look upon the positive. This afternoon at approximately 3:22 P.M. Eastern, the space capsule is scheduled to take off. The hours leading up to the liftoff will be exciting. We have already been told that this launch is the first from American soil in ten years. Let us pray for a successful mission and that our astronauts remain safe. But now, I have a pool to clean, birds, chipmunks and squirrel to feed and my wife said something about chores I should finish. I wonder what she means.

In the three and a half hours between now and the launch of the Crew Dragon space capsule, there seems to be a lessening of interest in the recording of deaths from COVID-19. That's a good thing; morbidity is unhealthy. And, it's the weekend. Main-desk media anchors are at home in high-rise Manhattan apartments or in big homes on Long Island or in New Jersey. Everyone needs some time off. Most of the news has to do with cancellations of sporting events, concerts, celebrations and store closings. Some governors still have not given approval to those wanting to get out and work. My guess is that the weekend guys are in Minneapolis hoping for a scoop.

Will today's launch in Florida be successful? If it is, what a great shot in the arm it could be. Americans need some positive news. We shall see. While waiting for the historic liftoff, I am reminded that the launch site has been historic long before any fossil-fueled rockets took off from that area.

Everyone is familiar with the famous French writer, Jules Verne and his "Twenty Thousand Leagues Under the Sea" and "Around the World in Eighty Days". But among his other twenty books is "From the Earth to the Moon", a mid nineteenth-century novel. In that book, Verne's hero decides to send a rocket to the moon using a giant cannon. As a launching site, the antagonist chooses a place in Florida which we now call Cape Canaveral. Who'd a thunk it?

One hour until launch. What would you hope for? A meticulously-planned and precise countdown? Huge crowds watching from a distance? Not today (social distancing). Great numbers watching the T.V. coverage? Red, white and blue banners commemorating the American venture? The entire American media's approval? How about two out of three? Politics must play a role here. Let's hope for all good things and forget that 19 thing and social unrest…at least for an hour.

Eighteen minutes until launch. Weather looks good. Large crowds on Coco Beach and on nearby bridges can be seen. No social distancing here. Nobody is worried about the virus; something good is taking place, at least in Florida. As we wait for the ignition of the rocket to take place, I think back to past launches. I erroneously thought the rocket's trajectory would take it south toward South America. Not so. The rocket will head north along the Atlantic coast. Fourteen minutes…two minutes! Thirty seconds! 8, 7, 6, 5…It's off!

It is unfortunate that my ability to appropriately relate emotions at this point is lacking. To say that a feeling of pride in country is present does not adequately define what is going through my thoughts. It is something that few other countries and peoples are incapable of doing. It is the Stars and Stripes lifting peoples' hopes and dreams, and I am witness to it all. The launch is fault free, and two astronauts are on their way through space. But, in other places and cities in the United States, there is turmoil, looting and burning.

God's speed, Crew Dragon!

Disgust, revulsion, repugnance, distaste, nausea, abhorrence, loathing, contempt, outrage! Pick one. Any one of the above sums up the riots in our cities. But first, something needs to be said.

After yesterday's launch of Crew Dragon's rocket from Cape Canaveral, we had a continuous T.V. coverage of the protests against the gruesome killing of a black American. Earlier in most American cities, at least while the sun was shining, protesters were almost peaceful. However, as the day progressed and the sun began to set, police and public vehicles were burned, and human cockroaches crawled out of hiding and used the darkness to cloak their civil disobedience.

The United States has had riots in the past. Those riots have been terrible. However, the latest disruptions are beyond the pall of human decency. I have never seen so many raised middle fingers thrust into the onlooking camera lenses of the media. Knowing that the whole world was watching such of an out-of-control mob mentality was morally sickening, and it makes most Americans, those at home sheltering themselves and social distancing themselves from what might soon be a fictitious illness, feel shame. A disgusting stain now covers both rioters, the governors of many states, and the mayors of our cities. Even the city of Albany, a rural community in upstate New York, was caught up in this terrible chapter of American history. Protesters, their arms in the air, gave the impression of being peaceful bystanders. Not so. What they were doing was providing a screen between the police and the insurgents behind them who lobbed bottles, bricks and stones at the police. Peaceful indeed! There were no innocent bystanders today.

Have we forgotten the virus? Recently, a report has come out stating that since the beginning of the pandemic, if a person died of a pre-conditioned illness (cancer, heart disease, asthma, COPD), and that person had tested positive for the virus, the death certificate was to read, "Death by COVID-19". It is beginning to look more and more like some kind of contrived scheme to inflict harm on or to control the general population and the economy of the country. Could that be the case? Of course not. We don't believe in conspiracies. But it is time for the cities' mayors and the States' governors to take back the country from the anarchists now in control. Let's get on with it by first quelling the violence in the streets and turning those streets into walkways and places where businesses operate without handed-down restrictions.

JUNE 1, 2020

OK, reader, where do we go from here? We, fellow Americans, are in the midst of a pandemic, embroiled in race riots and the Southeast is now in the beginning of the hurricane season. Last night's demonstrations, lootings and burning of public property set a new low on the American scene. The only shining light at the moment was Saturday's successful launch of two astronauts into space and a successful docking with the International Space Station. In a T.V. interview with the two newest members of the space station, both men expressed their pride in the endeavor. That was good to see. But it does seem that such things take a back seat to the negativity driving the bus.

Last night in the Nation's Capital, mobs took to the street and did what mobs do—rampage, burn and destroy. Unruly crowds tried to storm the White House but were repelled by National Guard, police and Secret Service personnel. The President was taken immediately to the underground bunker for his safety, but the mob continued on to the next block and caused major damage. In New York City, Mayor de Blasio's daughter was taken into custody for breaking curfew and being in an area that had been looted. Other cities throughout the country suffered the same indignations.

What will happen this evening? Talks are taking place this morning with black American community members and religious leaders in an effort to resolve the problem. However, many are waiting for a definitive decision on the policeman who murdered George Floyd. Will curfews be broken again this evening? Will civility return to the streets? Unlikely. It has been reported that automobiles are being driven without plates to avoid identification. One car with Arizona plates was stopped and its occupants searched. Looted items were found in the car. The nihilist organization Antifa has been scrutinized and is under investigation. There is very little mention of this left-leaning group on media reports. Watching such despicable actions weakens one's resolve, but I have a suggestion.

This dark period of time reminds me of what Americans must have been going through in the early years of WWII. Americans were dying at a rate of almost 10,000 a day. Men and machines were burning and left like carrion along roadsides and in fields. We are now faced with three uncertainties: pestilence, civil unrest and nature's threat of hurricanes. But, you know, there just might be something which would not end the violence and mayhem, but would lower the ignition temperature of mob mentality.

—OK, Allen, what makes you think you know so much?

—Just listen. What are we now missing from our daily lives that we had just four months ago?

—How should I know? You tell me.

—Sure. We had music. We had amphitheaters packed with fans not holding up placards saying, "Kill the white folks" and "Black lives matter". They were holding up cell-phone lights and weaving and waving to the beat of some pop-tune idol. They would sing along with the lyrics thinking that they, too, would drive off later in exotic limousines and fly off to some remote island in the Caribbean. Americans would travel great distances to see their favorite musicians and pay enormous sums just to spend a few hours in the fantasy of being close to stardom.

—So, how do we know that this might work, and how would it take place?

—Easy. Cordon off the main city blocks in our major cities. Times Square, for example. With the government's help, pay the rock stars to perform and charge nothing for these open-air concerts. Use the proceeds to help set up commissions on investigating how to improve race relations. Call these concerts, "A Way to Peace Through George Floyd".

—Sounds stupid.

—I think you are forgetting that I graduated in the top ten of my high-school class. It was a small school though.

Upended! Just like the high-end fashion-store mannequins in New York City's elite shopping centers, COVID-19 has been shoved aside and is taking second place in the news. Rioters, looters and burners have taken over the number one spot. Our cities' mayors seem to be helping the black-clad mob members by setting the curfew for 11 P.M. What? I'm in bed by 9, and the curfew is at 11? Nice move. Governors in many states are against a strong crackdown on the devastation taking place in their cities. I wonder why. In New York State, Governor Cuomo is no longer complaining about not enough ventilators, not enough PPE's and not enough hospital beds. He has other problems. So do we. But some things have not changed. The rioters are still wearing masks but for the wrong reason. Hard to tell who is who.

In a Phoenix Magazine article dating back to April, a column was devoted to shop owners who were facing shutdowns of their businesses. Among their concerns was the obligation to their employees. Everyone has bills. Mortgages, rent, credit card overages and other vital purchases must be handled. Some restaurant owners emptied their pantries by giving workers and the Salvation Army donations of food. That was two months ago. Some of those shops in Tempe and in the surrounding area of Phoenix no longer have store fronts. They have been burned out or looted. We are swiftly approaching the time when active military units might have to be called in to restore order. The United States is now at war.

At this point in my writing, I now wonder whether anything will be done by our elected officials. Whether it is a community organizer, councilman, mayor, governor, member of Congress or the President, we are in need of a strong response to the mayhem taking place on our streets. Will we get it tonight? Not with curfews set at 11 P.M. We will have a better idea at sunset or soon after.

This afternoon, the city coroner in Minneapolis and Dr. Michael Baden, a well-known pathologist, confirmed that George Floyd died of asphyxia. That fact points at premeditation and could lead to charges of murder in the first degree. That declaration, however, has not stopped the threat of more violence. Last night, one of the protesters stood in front of a media camera and shouted, "And, tonight, we're coming into your small neighborhood and going into your house and taking what's ours!" Now, such a threat might not be a good idea where I live. In upstate New York, two hundred thousand deer hunters with enough ammunition to last for months are waiting for 'deer season' to begin. Me, I don't hunt. But, yes, my Glock and my M1 Carbine are locked and loaded. How has it come to such a place?

It is now rumored that outside elements like Antifa have helped stir and agitate the protesters. Some police officers are now taking a knee and marching in support of the groups who allegedly are showing remorse for Floyd. One person, the niece of Martin Luther Jr. used her uncle's words to try to bring sense to the situation, "We may have come to America on different ships, but we are in the same boat now." I hope it stays afloat.

Riots, autopsies, looting, and despair dot this morning's news. Yesterday, Macy's Flagship and luxury store in New York City was looted. Police officers were under attack and one officer in another American city was shot but will recover. Mayor De Blasio's daughter was one of the agitators in yesterday's violence, and she was arrested. Her father, the New York City Mayor, praised his daughter saying that he was proud that she did the right thing in protesting police brutality. She was not charged with breaking any law. In the mayor's city, over 100 rioters were arrested in Sunday's violence and immediately released. Reminds me of fishing ventures. That will teach them! Four more cops were shot in St. Louis. The starkness, annoyance and despondency are working themselves into the American psyche. What other terrible news will be recorded today?

The virus, social distancing and sheltering-in-place have disappeared in the smoke of burning shops and places of business. The President has threatened to call in the National Guard if necessary. But Democrat governors around the country are against that idea. Surprising. Well, not really. Some members of Congress are blaming the social unrest on the President. Surprising. Other exasperated Americans are now arming themselves and seem to be ready to exercise their Second Amendment rights. My Glock? Right where it should be—close.

This morning, *Madame et moi* played a couple games of pickle ball. The fact that I am able to play the game at my age is not important. But, today, phase 2 in Governor Cuomo's plan to open up the economy is beginning to take shape, and ball courts are in that plan. I played only two games. Hey, as I just said, age limits things. Let me wager that because everyone is now openly flaunting the social distancing rule in the streets with impunity, more and more places of business will open up. Let's see what the rest of the day brings.

The war continues. Not against the virus, but against each other. Every war, and we are in a war, claims lives and property. WWII (39-45) produced 66 million dead, and nearly 70 percent—some 46 million—were civilians according to information furnished by National Graphic Magazine. Civilians are again taking the brunt of the burden and grief in this war against the pandemic and racism. What might it take to get the attention of our law-abiding citizens? We hesitate to suggest vigilantism, but it might indeed take an outpouring of physical presence and verbal condemnation of this wholesale violence. Those on the left have criticized the Americans who protested in front of Michigan's capital building while carrying AR-15's. But those protesters did not fire a shot. No one was killed. Contrast that with the street riots in other cities. Politics? Ah, would it not be nice if we could abolish political affiliation until we came up with an effective vaccine?

—Wait! We might never come up with a vaccine.
—My point exactly!

In this morning's news, many American cities are cleaning up after last night's curfews were broken and the rampage ended. In Washington, a special unit of swat-trained officers was on the street at 8 A.M. No rioters, looters or protesters were in sight. But it does make one wonder why we would have riot busters on the streets when no one else was present. Rioters sleep till noon. They come out at night like vampires when the sun goes down. I wonder who writes the "Quelling a Riot" book.

"Stay safe!" is an expression which no longer means, wear a mask, social distance yourself and shelter-in-place. Stay safe now means, stay out of the way of rioters. You could get hurt. Another word needs clarification, too. "Transparency" is the new watch word used by elected officials and media. It is hard to understand how we are to define a word which has never been clarified. Some of us see through the ruse, however.

President Trump is being highly criticized for having suggested that the National Guard and certain military units be used in response to the looting. "Too harsh" yell the media and some of the President's staff. On the other hand, Joe Biden recently suggested that the police shoot the rioters in the leg and not in the heart. No immediate condemnation from either the media or political colleagues. Hum? But Biden later apologized for his remarks. All forgiven.

In a morning Fox News report, an anchor asked Senator John Kennedy from Louisiana why President Trump was criticized for his posing with a Bible in front of an historic Washington church. Kennedy's response was classic home-spun irony. He said, "Here's a newsflash for you. Some people in Washington don't like Trump." In my experience with Trump haters, there are two statements that drip off their tongues immediately when asked why they hate the President" He lies and he is a racist. Those subjective comments are never backed up with evidence and they ring hollow from being trite and overused. But let's move on to something personal and positive.

In the midst of all this anarchy, someone somewhere made a good decision. My granddaughter, Marley, a senior in high school, had been working in a local restaurant on weekends and in the summers. When COVID-19 led to the closing of restaurants and places of businesses in March, Marley's money for college dried up. Recently, however, this enterprising young lady was informed that she would be receiving $600.00 a week in unemployment benefits until the fall when she matriculated at university. Whoever initiated that law had foresight. But we still are facing strife on the home front.

The chances are good that the violence in our streets has not ended. The fact that we are in a presidential-election year does not help. Good or bad, whatever is decided in the way of bringing us out or this maelstrom of disillusionment would be a godsend. I might even give up playing pickle ball. No way! I've been through tougher things. So have you. Let's beat back both the pandemic and the hatred.

Overnight in New York City, members of the NYPD were ambushed. Two police officers were shot, and one was stabbed in the neck by a curfew breaker who approached the officers from behind. In many other American cities, similar attacks on the police took place. T.V. coverage of this morning's cleanup showed city workers picking up blue plastic containers filled with bricks and stones. Such containers were brought in by rioters and deposed in crucial areas and intersections in preparation for another round of mayhem. No one seems able or willing to identify the suppliers of these lethal weapons.

Black against white, white against black has not subsided. One well-to-do neighborhood in Maryland organized a group of affluent white homeowners and encouraged them to kneel on the ground and apologize for their white privilege. Cute! I have yet to take a knee in support of what some other American has down against any other person. But, an NFL player, Drew Brees openly stated that he would never take a knee during the playing of the National Anthem. He was later criticized by fellow black players for being insensitive to the issue at hand. He immediately apologized and retracted his previous statement. Diversity? Maybe not.

Ah, what the Hell. Here's another personal anecdote. Being born and brought up in Western Pennsylvania in the 40's and 50's meant that my family were hard working coal miners and tannery employees. Tough people. In our little Susquehanna River town, minorities were just that—few in number. But those were not Caucasian, worked just as hard as any others in the community, and they believed in God. "So what?", you say. Well, none of them would have crept up on you from behind and stabbed you in the neck. On my high-school football team, we had an especially accomplished running back. He was black, and I was his main blocker. I thought highly of him then. I still do, and I never thought anything but praise when I welcomed him back across the goal line after he had made a touchdown. Later, as a Marine, I shared foxholes with black-American Marines, and that made me proud; we were together. Later, when working as a teacher, some of my students were black Americans, and one family's parent, the father, was a former Tuskegee Airman whom I greatly admired. He flew P-51 Mustangs over Italy and was shot down twice before he came home, went to school and became an engineer at GE. While I revere my association with such people, I will never get down on my knee and apologize for being who I am. You shouldn't either. Now, let's get on with it.

There is now a warning that those who took part in the riots and protests might have contributed to a second wave of the virus. After all, no social distancing took place, and the rioters sure as Hell were not sheltering-in-place. The media is quick to add that teargas makes one cough. No kidding! I have experienced it in Marine training. I didn't cough, but breathing was difficult. Will we have another round of shop closings, pleas for PPE's from governors who whined incessantly for everything imaginable and then chose not to use them? We might have to wait until July to tell; you know, the fourteen-day thing. But, for one, I am tired of governors who want to keep America closed down. Why should thousands of out-of-control youth be encouraged to march in protest hand-in-hand and shop owners forced to fend for themselves while their businesses remain closed? That oxymoron must be addressed. Let's see what the day brings.

News flash! Herschel Walker, a Heisman Trophy Winner and former NFL player questioned his own race about their penchant for disruption and looting. He agreed that protests were appropriate, but he wondered why anyone would condone the burning and looting of community property. Herschel, you will be chastised for your standing up against stupidity.

In Scottsdale, AZ yesterday, a young You-Tube producer and performer was arrested in a looting incident at Fashion Square, an upscale shopping area. His defense was given as he was just taking pictures of others who were breaking windows and looting merchandise. Innocent, I say. Huh? I do wonder what the last remaining members of the Greatest Generation would think of the young people now tearing down what they fought to protect. I think you know... don't you.

Every sort of unimaginable thing is now taking place in and around America. Our most well-known bigot and racist, Al Sharpton, just delivered the eulogy for George Floyd at a funeral ceremony. That Sharpton, a guy who, when he lived in New York City, would hire school bus drivers to drive him and fifty or sixty others to job sites, and when there, would get off and shake down the clerk of the works by stating that if blacks were not hired, he would protest. That threat would give Sharpton $500.00 to $1,000.00 on the spot. Sharpton and his busload of potential work stoppers would continue on the next site, and at noon, the busload of people would be dropped off at McDonalds where Sharpton would buy lunch. Now, that same shakedown artist is an anchor at MSNBC where he is considered to be the spokesperson for right and wrong. From where does this information come? A young former Marine was working the same sites trying to sell Rawl Plug tools to the same clerk of the works. The seller was Brooks Remaley.

Officials in Minneapolis and in New York City, have called for the defunding of their police departments. White men and women are now asked to get down on both knees and renounce their 'whiteness' and atone for their sins.

In Bethesda, MD, a large group of affluent homeowners did just that in a great display of righteousness. Groups of protesters armed with all the tools necessary (crowbars, hammers and axes) are now getting ready for curfew hour which will provide cover for their acts of violence. More police officers across the country were killed and maimed yesterday.

In the fifth century A.D., the city of Rome was sacked and burned. Its sacred sites were burned and looted by the Vandals, an out-of-control Germanic tribe. We now have our own vandals, and they are wreaking havoc on our city streets. Some Americans are calling for someone in authority to invoke the 'Military Powers Act' and clear the streets of an invading force. "Too harsh!", say those in city halls. Why? Good question. However, it looks more and more like some Americans who would like to see things get worse. Makes for a more-level voting opportunity in November.

When will this chronicle of events end? Some predict that a successful vaccine against the virus might do it. I don't think so. Once the taste of blood is in the water, scavengers rise to the surface. Is this an urge to inflict vengeance and threaten a defenseless public? The Governor of the State of Virginia, a man who once dressed himself in blackface to celebrate a university graduation, has just announced that his state is taking down the statue of Robert E. Lee. I wonder if those dead now resting on Lee's former property in Arlington Cemetery are turning over in their graves.

If I am ever asked by either my children of by my grandchildren what I think of such strife going on around me, I would tell them this: When you have time, look into the lives of at least twenty great Americans who have contributed to the welfare and growth of this county we call home. Ask yourselves what it was that made men storm the beaches at Normandy and at Iwo Jima knowing that they might never see the light of another day. Ask yourselves what made a black woman in the rear of a bus take a front seat along with others. Then, once you have an idea of the reasons why people did good things, emulate their efforts. I would tell my family members to be proud of who they are, to avoid skin color when trying to evaluate the good and the bad of a fellow American. I would tell them, those of my blood, to respect the flag, to honor it and to never bend a knee in support of a presupposed new way of thinking. I would advise my family members to work toward the belief in a God who offers a salvation and encourages the best of each person. You do what you want. I'll do my part, too.

Yesterday afternoon, I witnessed a blatant act of insensitivity. In Buffalo, NY, the police were in the act of clearing pedestrians from the streets. A seventy-eight-year-old man was in the way. Either because of his age and/or his inability to hear, the man hesitated and was pushed backward. He stumbled, fell and cracked open his skull on the hard pavement. That, ladies and gentlemen, was police brutality. Little was said about the incident on media reports. The man was white. Let's see how much coverage this is given in today's broadcasts. Oh, by the way. Today is the anniversary of the Invasion of Normandy where 10,000 Americans lost their lives on the first day. Will that event be covered in today's news? Check it out.

Transparency, systemic racism, defunding, some lives matter, remain in lockdown, upon up the economy, vandalism, N95 masks and all the other invented, overused and subtle efforts to explain the early months of 2020. It borders on nausea. And here we are in another weekend. The repeat of last week's happenings will be served up by the media as if it makes sense to them. They will opine instead of reporting about the disgusting scenes of rampage and looting in our streets. Thousands of people holding signs saying, "Black Lives Matter", "No justice, no peace.", "George Floyd lives.", and the new one, "Defund the police." On that last sign, some cities such as Minneapolis and Los Angeles are proposing just that. A new system having to do with community organizers running departments of public safety. Imagine what that might be like. No describe it to someone in dire need of assistance telling them, just use your cell phone. "Who ya gonna call?"

Where is the virus in all this wave of violence? It's hiding. Was it scared off by all the bull-horn voices and fireworks? Seems so. Many people are still wearing masks, but I think that keeping those face coverings is more a fashion statement than a health aid. Yesterday, there was a bit of good news, i.e., if you want stability and an upward spiral of the economy. There was a drop in unemployment and the figures on Wall Street rose. In some states, phase 2 of the opening was taking place. Could this be the beginning of a recovery? Hard to tell. Health-care analysists are still wondering whether a second wave of COVID-19 will occur because of so many protesters not following the social distancing laws. We will know in about two weeks, the period of time it takes for testing positive to the contagion.

Looking back over the massive gatherings of those in support of this or that, I have a question. Where are all these young adults coming from, and how do they have so much time on their hands? Wait. I know the answer to that question. In March we shut down our schools and universities. We have refused to reopen them, and are reluctant to give a time when they might again turn lights on in classrooms. Hundreds of thousands of students, all of working age, are now living at home during the day and patrolling the streets from 4 P. M. to 4 A.M. "Mom, I'm home!" Before leaving that place of security, those young people might say, "Let's march in protest. Let's show solidarity with those who are oppressed. Hey, there's merchandise in those stores. Anyone got a crowbar?" OK, just funnin'. Unfortunately, our careless decision of closing certain institutions of learning has created monsters. If there is any one decision in the coming weeks which is important, it hinges on our schools. They should be reopened, and soon.

As a former educator, I must wonder what today's classroom professors and teachers are telling our students. There is evidence that left-wing college teachers, the progressives and the minimalists, are encouraging their students to disrespect the rule of law. Hey, these students are of the age when they could volunteer for military service. Don't think that is likely. But there is no need to lose respect for those who did wear the uniform…the military uniform. Seems like the color blue is unpopular…until you need them, of course.

You know, there comes a time when you have seen enough. The events of the past three months make one wish for a renewal, a fresh look. At the same time, we would like to see more Americans respect the past. God, family, country. We, or at least some of us, should remain vigilant and walk our posts in a military manner, and if called upon to add sense to mayhem, we should step forward.

I do not know what the outcome of all this sound and fury will be. If I were to predict that our country would not only survive but be better than ever, some would chide me for being too Trump-like. That would not disturb me. I'm not going down on one knee. But let's hope that July, August, September and October bring opportunities for hope and happiness. The only people who can bring that about is us, Americans of every color, race and ethnicity. Why not?

ENDGAME

In the game of chess, there comes a time when the major redaction of forces has taken place. Decisions have to be made at such a point. It is time for me to get away from all the madness. It is debilitating, and I need my strength for pickle ball and banjo playing. Everything comes to an end. It is my sincere hope that this pandemic burns itself out, that some miraculous vaccine is discovered which destroys all types of corona…not the beer, of course. It is my hope that all Americans, every one of us, realize that life and the gift of being able to enjoy every second of it is fleeting. Racial turmoil is a senseless waste of precious time and energy.

It is my hope that the reader of this short tome realizes that his opinion of my thoughts has no weight. Don't even think about it. That's another waste of time. I give credit to my grandson, Mackinley Hawthorne, and my granddaughter, Marley Hawthorne, for their rendition the cover of 19. Oh, if you found any misspelled words, Marilyn did it.

Let me hope that you read this on one of the front pages of your favorite newspapers: 'Eighty-one-year-old former teacher and former Marine comes up with a magnificent vaccine. The vaccine does not cure or prevent any form of a coronavirus, but it does rid the country of a biased media and it wipes out racial intolerance. On sale at your local pharmacy for $39.95.'

FIN

POSTSCRIPT

It is perhaps uncommon that an afterthought might be included at the end of a manuscript. But sometimes, it is needed. If there is anything learned in my recording of the events of the last three months, it is this: we know now that in this world of immense beauty and astonishing wonder, we will encounter a few people who do not see. Their view of others is distorted by abuse from those around them, from having had the wrong environment during their formative years, or from having been the victim of intolerance. Some things are unavoidable. In the end, however, once the dust has settled from the stomping of feet on the dried-up mud of broken things, there is still the chance, one more opportunity, for clarity. Ask those around you to describe the beauty they see. Depending on their description of how they interpret life and your understanding of their point of view, there still might be hope.

As of today's date, and since February of this year, over 110,000 Americans have succumbed to 19.

06/07/2020
Saratoga Springs, NY

AFTERTHOUGHT

Something just does not smell right in all this. Seeping out from under the flotsam of the past four months, there is a foul-smelling stench. Put in this devil's mix a supposedly lethal and stealth-like virus—an escapee from some little-known secret lab in some far-off country. Thousands of unsuspecting carriers of this contagion spread the disease unknowingly to millions of others throughout the world. Add to this noxious concoction a gruesome murder of a man of color, and stir this brew in the streets of our major cities. Let it warm up over the fires of discontent fanned by an over-zealous media and political opportunists. Now, as a backdrop, paint the portrait of one of the best-performing economies in decades. Step back, and look at the picture. Ask yourselves, could all this have been contrived in some back room by a few people who wanted change? Nah! That's not possible. It's too much like…

June 10, 2020